The Inner Fitness Revolution

Also by Tina Lifford

The Little Book of Big Lies

THE
INNER FITNESS
REVOLUTION

A Roadmap to Your Freedom and Joy

———

Tina Lifford

AMISTAD

An Imprint of HarperCollins*Publishers*

THE INNER FITNESS REVOLUTION. Copyright © 2025 by Dare to Ask, Inc. All rights reserved. Printed in the United States of America. No part of this book may be used or reproduced in any manner whatsoever without written permission except in the case of brief quotations embodied in critical articles and reviews. For information, address HarperCollins Publishers, 195 Broadway, New York, NY 10007.

HarperCollins books may be purchased for educational, business, or sales promotional use. For information, please email the Special Markets Department at SPsales@harpercollins.com.

FIRST EDITION

Designed by Yvonne Chan
Circle art throughout © Yuliia Borovyk/stock.adobe.com
Blocks icon used throughout © Iconic Prototype/stock.adobe.com
Illustration on page 2 © rost9/stock.adobe.com
Illustration on page 43 © alekseyvanin/stock.adobe.com
Illustration on page 55 © Mary Long/stock.adobe.com
Thought bubble on page 55 © yuruphoto/stock.adobe.com

Library of Congress Cataloging-in-Publication Data has been applied for.

ISBN 978-0-06-293031-6

24 25 26 27 28 LBC 5 4 3 2 1

To Mommy

and

To the inner Self that can guide and support our every step.

Contents

Preface

I'M TINA LIFFORD, AND I WELCOME YOU TO THE INNER FIT-ness Revolution.

Worldwide, people are waking up to their innate right to feel better, do better, and be better in life. They are saying "no" to running from the past, caving to insecurity, and seeing hurt, bad parenting, trauma, and ignorance as a life sentence. Legions of internal freedom seekers are challenging the tyranny of unhelpful thoughts, feelings, and beliefs that overwhelm and restrict their thriving.

The Self inside you is more powerful than the tyranny, and your innate purpose is undeniable. You are the answer to every problem and desire in your life, and you are born to thrive.

In your hands is a roadmap to greater internal freedom and wellbeing. This revolutionary journey marches you unapologetically across the plains of the past into an empowered, loving, compassionate, honest, committed, and empathetic relationship with your Self.

For more than thirty years, my mission—first in my personal life and now in the world as the founder of the Inner Fitness Project—has been to make **inner fitness** as well-understood and actionable as physical fitness.

You might know me from my thirty years as a working actress: In the 1990s I played Joan Mosley in the television series *South*

Central, Mama Haze in *The Temptations*, and Winnie Mandela opposite Sidney Poitier in the movie *Mandela and de Klerk*; in 2002 I starred with Clint Eastwood in *Blood Work*, and in 2005 with Bruce Willis in *Hostage*. From 2010 to 2015, I played Renee Trussell in the television series *Parenthood*. From 2015 to 2017, I played CIA Director Lowry in *Scandal*. Most recently, I played Aunt Vi in the critically acclaimed series *Queen Sugar* on the Oprah Winfrey Network for seven seasons. I've played more than a hundred characters from my start in community theater. I am passionate about bringing characters to life. I am even more passionate about inner fitness and bringing more aliveness to the lives of real people. This is the work I have the honor of doing at the Inner Fitness Project. "Inner fitness" supports inner wellbeing—your mental, emotional, and spiritual states.

We know that physical fitness strengthens the body and supports wellness. However, **wellness and wellbeing are not the same**. Wellness addresses the physical body, while wellbeing benefits the Self *inside* the body—the health of our thoughts, feelings, and beliefs and the actions and reactions they cause.

Physical exercise strengthens the body against physical challenges and supports clearer thinking, relieves the stress of managing internal dis-ease, helps us look great, unleashes endorphins that elevate our mood briefly, and momentarily *distracts* us from feeling overwhelmed by our deeper unresolved issues. However, physical exercise does not resolve our internal problems—it does not reorder our thinking, eliminate feelings of inadequacy or unworthiness, or make us emotionally resilient in the long term. Physical exercise does not administer forgiveness, assuage guilt and shame, or help us navigate loss, anxiety, or disconnection from ourselves.

Here's an analogy I use in my workshops: *The physical body is the vehicle, and the inner Self drives the car.*

Most people live life trying to be the right vehicle: They dress and speak well, say the right things, aim to be important, and make a lot of money. Yet, they suffer internally because they do not know they are more than their past hurts, their negative isolating thoughts, or their bank accounts.

It is time to stop living life on the basis of appearances and perceptions. We must stop stepping over our inner Self and allowing our internal issues and pasts to dictate our lives. We must discover we are more than our deepest wounds and challenges and begin to prioritize valuing and strengthening the inner Self.

Developing a strong inner Self leads to a healthier internal state and greater Self-awareness and freedom. This effort is nothing short of a revolution.

By turning our focus to our thoughts, feelings, and beliefs, we are arming ourselves with mental health awareness, marching into therapists' offices, and saying "no more" to ignoring the inner Self.

Inner fitness strategies are powerful practices that improve wellbeing by promoting Self-discovery, Self-awareness, Self-acceptance, and Self-love.

With inner fitness, you condition your internal response to life. You learn and practice the ability to guide your thinking and disrupt your ingrained negativity biases by using simple tools, such as *shifting your attention*, *sitting in your observer's chair*, and *following this book's 14 Practices for Inner Health and Wellbeing*. You navigate difficulty and practice Self-awareness, focused on positive possibilities and thriving more than surviving.

Therapy and inner fitness work are not mutually exclusive but can be combined to create a powerful journey of Self-improvement. By incorporating one or both into your life, you engage in a transformative process that leads to a better version of YOU.

As an inner fitness practitioner for more than three decades, I am "practiced" at navigating life consciously engaged with my inner Self. My sleeves have been rolled up, and I have been working my inner awareness through trial and error—even before it became fashionable to do so.

As the founder of the Inner Fitness Project, I strive to demystify inner work and identify effective internal practices that we can default to as readily as we engage physical fitness exercises.

An Inner Fitness Case Study

The 2020 COVID pandemic allowed me time to focus on establishing an online presence for the Inner Fitness Project and the Inner Fitness Studio. At the studio I teach inner fitness mindsets and exercises I have gathered, created, and practiced for decades. The common sense and ease of use behind inner fitness resonated with people. My programs changed lives. Some transformations were dramatic. People grieving or feeling lost or out of alignment with themselves for years experienced profound shifts in just seven days. Awareness of the inner Self and respect for Self-care were enhanced greatly for many. These early case studies proved that regular engagement with inner fitness practices was as beneficial as physical fitness to the health of individuals and, therefore, to families and the world. Participants began to engage their lives with a life-enhancing sense of accountability to themselves. They reported experiencing elevated moods, an exciting sense of possibility, and increased internal comfort almost immediately. Many participants said they continued to grow as they practiced inner fitness strategies. The openness and trust that emerged turned the Inner Fitness Studio into a community where people feel safe, seen, and heard and have come to the comforting realization that their personal challenges are a testament to the human experience.

The Inner Fitness Project is revolutionary in presenting systematic, proactive inner Self-care, including the **14 Practices for Inner Health and Wellbeing** on page 81 that are at the core of this book.

Though mental and emotional overwhelm appears to be the new normal, we can disrupt that trajectory in our personal lives and positively impact society's future. This belief gets me up in the morning and lives at the core of everything we do at the Inner Fitness Project.

TheInnerFitnessProject.com

The Inner Fitness Project is a wellbeing movement and community. On our website, you will find information, shared experiences, and programs that have helped others change their lives. I welcome you to visit the Inner Fitness Project and check out our studio, join our mailing list, and download any worksheets or material mentioned in this book. Add your passion to the Inner Fitness Revolution, and let's stand side by side in this wellbeing revolution and give one another permission to be well. Visit www.TheInnerFitnessProject.com.

Introduction

WHEN PEOPLE ASK ME WHAT I DO WHEN I AM NOT ACT-ing, I say, "I help people discover and strengthen their inner Self." When people hear this, they are intrigued.

The inner Self comprises your thoughts, feelings, beliefs, actions, and reactions, and strengthens the ability to act in your mental, emotional, and spiritual best interest in any circumstance. I call this work *inner fitness*. **Inner fitness develops skills and practices that build mental, emotional, and spiritual strength and resilience.**

I come to this work with a fire in my belly and love in my heart. Discovering your inner Self is the new frontier. Can't you feel it in the air? Though philosophers, monks and nuns, spiritual leaders, and mystics have walked this road for thousands of years, today's collective human pain and discontent demand a more resonating conversation. We must adopt new beliefs and actions. People yearn to feel better and to know, trust, and honor themselves. This desire for Self-connection is an exciting advent in our human development. It helps us see a correlation between how we think, feel, and believe, and how we relate to ourselves and act or react in the world.

Many people resist Self-discovery because they are terrified of looking inside themselves and discovering they are broken and unworthy. But we are learning that trauma, misinformation, and lies have played a role in our fear and distrust of ourselves. Neuroscience, human potential research, and spirituality are helping us see ourselves more accurately and transform our judgment of ourselves into informed insights. Instead of seeing ourselves as broken or not good enough, we can use science and spirituality to see our strengths, cultivate resilience, have compassion for ourselves and the human experience, and foster genuine admiration and respect for Self.

Revolutions seek desired change. A more enlightened, respectful, honest, and trusting relationship with their inner Self awaits anyone who wants it. The insights and practices in this book will usher in profound Self-appreciation and Self-respect. To this end, throughout the book, *Self* is mostly spelled with a capital *S* to practice assigning respect to the word instead of seeing it merely as tacked onto the back of other words such as *myself, yourself, herself,* or *himself* like a caboose. Too often, the inner Self is overlooked, seen as a villain or victim, the cause of pain and shame rather than the supporter and creative instrument the Self can be.

By reading this book, you can acknowledge and challenge your limiting beliefs and hurtful stories and embrace the hope that greater internal freedom is possible.

My Growth

In my personal development, I have attended countless workshops and trainings as either a student or facilitator and worked with private clients and corporations. I've heard the longings of thousands of people. The most common aches are the desire for a loving relationship or the hope of finding freedom from a painful experience. I was a student in those workshops because I was searching for tools for managing emotional overwhelm. Also, I'm an "old soul" and a truth seeker.

My first passion is being curious about living life well and seeking answers to emotional challenges. My other passion is acting—using my body and heart to understand and tell another person's story. These driving forces are intricately linked.

In my first book, *The Little Book of Big Lies*, I shared my fifth-grade trauma of freezing onstage before the entire student body during a schoolwide talent show. I was so lost in fear that my teacher had to carry me off the stage. That formative experience led me to a self-investigation that helped me discover there was more to me than my default insecurities, worries, and fears. As I matured, addressing that experience with compassion and courage has proved liberating. The adage that our greatest pain can be our greatest gift is true. When we use pain to grow, the benefit of increased Self-acceptance, capability, and emotional resilience gives us greater inner freedom and peace.

We all have fears and grievances that undermine our authentic Self. We must forgive ourselves for making some choices and permit ourselves to envision our dreams. Achieving these desires requires quality time with our Self, which will help us sort through our thoughts, discover outdated beliefs, and identify our assumptions, projections, limiting habits, and lies.

* * *

The key concepts, 14 Practices, and real-life stories I share in this book are the kind of EFFORT and quality time with your Self that will lead to a wiser, more whole Self. EFFORT isn't defined as hard work. At the Inner Fitness Project, **EFFORT** stands for Extracting Freedom From Our Restricted Thinking. We must learn to move beyond troubling experiences by extracting positive insights from them. The simple concepts in this book guide your EFFORT so that you can start thinking about and responding to life more positively.

Many philosophers and mystics say the answers to all our questions live inside us, waiting to be discovered and lived. But answers are like precious gems; we must mine them and hone them to bring their beauty into our lives.

Developing inner fitness can help us achieve the rewarding internal life we want—feeling capable of thriving beyond any storm, feeling known and understood, courageously living a life that is true to ourselves, transforming our relationship to our uncomfortable thoughts and past, turning self-doubt and judgment into self-acceptance, and living from a sense of purpose.

In this book I share transformational mindset tools and the Inner Fitness Project's **Three Selves** framework to help you understand the full range of your inner Self and navigate life with more intent and personal power. The 14 Practices will give you tools for addressing any life situation to feel empowered and aligned with your Self.

Every conscious EFFORT to support your inner Self is a revolutionary act.

Unfortunately, we are not taught to nurture the inner Self, nor to seek its truth. Managing the appearance of things in our lives is the norm. But through trial and error, I became aware of the inner Self and how necessary inner fitness is to growth and wellbeing. Everything I share in this book has proved invaluable in my personal journey. However, magically, the journey curates itself to each person. You will engage your tailor-made experience through prompts, speaking out loud, and exercises. The dictionary defines a "**journey**" as the act of traveling from one place to another. You will not be the same person at the end of your journey. You will find yourself in another place, and you will experience your own personal Revolution!

When you know your Self, you are empowered.
When you accept your Self, you are invincible.

My Vow to You

T HROUGH THIS JOURNEY TO BETTER UNDERSTAND YOUR Self you will discover that a healthy and rewarding relationship with your Self is possible and is rich in its depth. Also, you will love and honor your Self more.

Whether you are feeling broken, lost, stuck, or overwhelmed; whether you want to move into a new life chapter, are tired of beating yourself up or giving yourself away to everything and everyone in your life; or whether you want to stop living life as one big competition, soften your hardened heart, and trust life more—every imaginable constriction and problem will change for the better as you practice the art of becoming your whole Self. Yes, unwanted thoughts and feelings can overwhelm, steer, and control your mind, but you can learn to exercise more Self-agency over them.

Your revolutionary act is to know you are capable of creating the life you want and to cling to your right to feel better, do better, and be better.

Between this page and the last one in this book, you will learn that the power to move your life forward and be happier lives inside you already. Spoiler alert: *You are already whole.* What has been missing is understanding the nature of your Self and working with your Self more intentionally.

I encourage you to take your time. This is not a quick read but rather an opportunity to spend quality time with your Self. Allow the book to be a guide and a coach: read, contemplate, and engage with it like a conversation with a good friend.

On this journey, I use the word *we* as much as I use *you* because we each are navigating our version of the human journey with its similar struggles and joys, though our specific details vary. We are walking this road together. Let's cheer one another on. In this spirit, should you have questions on this revolutionary journey of reclaiming your Self, feel free to email them to support @theinnerfitnessproject.com.

Now, let's set you up for success by introducing a few guidelines and inner fitness tools you'll need for the journey ahead.

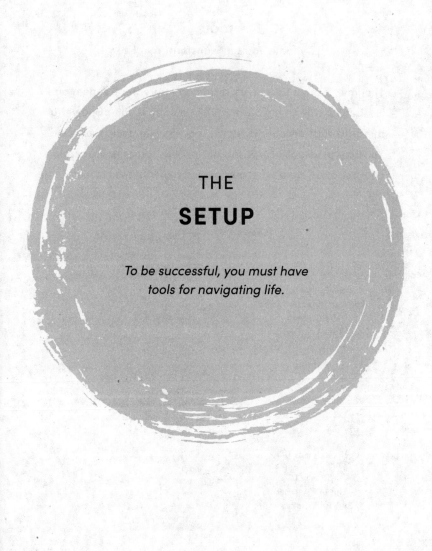

THE

SETUP

To be successful, you must have tools for navigating life.

TOOLS

Dynamic Tools to Transform Your Life

The Inner Fitness Revolution roadmap to greater freedom and joy begins wherever you are. This journey is full of powerful mindsets that become dynamic tools for enhancing your life. You'll be pleasantly surprised at how this roadmap generates new behavior. Here's the journey and benefits in a nutshell:

A New Sense of Self

7 Laws of Self
Talk to Your Self
Play More
Tell Your Self the Truth

Have an Intention
Let Your Inner Self Lead
Be Curious
Don't Take Life Personally

Up Until Now, That's How Life Has Been
Know Your Three Selves
Sit in Your Observer's Chair
Say "I See You" to the Past

Shift Your Focus
CREWW UP
The 14 Practices
Be Your Whole Self

The 7 Laws of Self

———

In any revolution, you must know that
what you are fighting for is worth it.

A N INTERNAL REVOLUTIONARY ACT IS ANY BEHAVIOR that supports and strengthens your inner Self.

The inner Self is worth the revolutionary act of challenging our inauthentic self to live authentically instead of pretending and performing. Too many of us tell ourselves hurtful stories about ourselves and drift away from our Self. Disconnection from our innate wholeness and worth occurs when we don't know, trust, or honor the Self.

The Inner Fitness Revolution, by definition, declares that *you have innate worth.* No person or choice you might make can rob you of this. Your worthiness is built into your DNA. Your work is to discover the truth of this statement and embody it—let it seep into your thoughts and guide your relationship with your Self.

Believing in your innate worth is easier said than done, for reasons that will become abundantly clear on this journey. Having the right tools and being armed with transformative insights will guide you. The more you can identify the behaviors that undermines the Self, the easier it is to see and believe that new behavior is possible.

> **Science Says**
>
> The latest neuroscience research says the brain has lifelong *plasticity*. This means the brain can change up to the day we take our last breath. No pain has to last forever. You can change how you view and interpret that pain.

* * *

I vividly remember the day my relationship with my Self changed forever. In 2005, when I was sitting in a spiritual psychology course, my professor said that events themselves are not the cause of unhappiness. Rather, unhappiness comes from how we think about ourselves as a result of the events we encounter.

As I scribbled this statement in my notebook, I found myself back in my hometown, watching Aunt Pang, my mother's good friend and my godmother, unravel. Aunt Pang became an alcoholic after she and Uncle Samuel divorced. I didn't understand then what I was seeing. Aunt Pang's downward slide scared me because all my young life, I had looked up to her.

My professor's statement explained Aunt Pang's demise: She saw herself as worthless. I realized that Aunt Pang's feelings of worthlessness began long before she met and married Uncle Samuel. She brought her learned feelings of worthlessness into her marriage.

Aunt Pang grew up during the 1930s. Her skin was shiny black. She was intelligent and beautiful. She made more money and had more social connections on both sides of the race line than almost anyone in the small town where she lived. But as a child, her shiny black color attracted relentless mean-spirited comments that seeped into her psyche. Inside the successful adult version of her was a deeply wounded child. She excelled in many areas partly because she was trying to outrun her negative view of herself.

When Aunt Pang met Uncle Samuel, a strikingly handsome man shades lighter than she was, they fell in love and married. He was devoted to her. But no one knew that Aunt Pang doubted her value and ability to be loved.

Often, Aunt Pang would offhandedly tell Uncle Samuel that he should find a girlfriend. One day, after many years of feeling that his love for her was being dismissed or minimized, he, in fact, found a girlfriend, divorced Aunt Pang, and married a woman who appreciated his commitment to her.

Losing Uncle Samuel left Aunt Pang devastated. But I believe her true pain and suffering stemmed from the deep-rooted idea she was unworthy. This had kept her from leaning in to and trusting Uncle Samuel's love for her, and was a reason she drank.

My professor's statement that events do not cause our unhappiness, but rather, unhappiness comes from how we think about ourselves because of our experiences, was a turning point. I wanted to spend my nonacting time living, and helping others live their lives, with keen Self-awareness and Self-respect.

* * *

Many people believe they are not good enough or, worse, that they are the problem. They are certain that the family they came from, the challenges they have faced, or the circumstances they have lived with are worse than what others experience. There are countless ways people see themselves as a problem. This Self-deprecating view is the major cause of suffering. Constantly seeing yourself as a problem and trying to fix yourself yet never succeeding is hell.

This is one reason the Inner Fitness Revolution is necessary: Seeing yourself as a problem is a misguided, pernicious belief that must be overthrown.

You are not a problem. You are the creative solution that can meet any problem that comes with life. You are powerful.

When we undermine, discount, abuse, reject, harshly judge, overlook, or dismiss ourselves, we tell ourselves we don't matter. This message is like poking holes in a water bucket, and our healthy sense of Self leaks out until we are empty. An empty bucket can't carry the water life needs to sustain itself. An empty Self becomes a bucket for anxiety, anger, dis-ease, and discontent, a life that never feels fully lived.

You must discover the Self that lives within you, understand that *your thoughts, feelings, and beliefs create your life*, and proactively strive to create a life that honors you.

Starting now, you can improve how you see and think about your Self in any situation. **The 7 Laws of Self** help you develop a respect-filled and thriving relationship with your Self. Laws are rules to live by that regulate our thoughts and behavior, and these 7 Laws will help you do that and guide your relationship with your Self. They are culled from the thousands of hours I've poured into studying psychology, spirituality, personal development, therapy, and working with or listening to thousands of people struggle with their negative stories about themselves.

Allow these 7 Laws to reset and govern how you see and talk to your Self. Let them remind you of your innate value, and cause you to treat your Self with more respect and compassion. Set a standard for how you see and engage with your Self:

Law 1: You have innate purpose and worth.

The goal: Stop trying to be "somebody" and instead be your wonderful, unique Self.

Law 2: The Self comprises your thoughts, feelings, and beliefs and creates your life's stories.

The goal: Adjust your thinking to interact with your Self more consciously and create your life more intentionally.

Law 3: A strong inner Self strengthens every area of your life.

The goal: Practice internal behavior that strengthens your relationship with your Self.

Law 4: You are connected to your higher power through the Self and can continually improve your life.

The goal: Learn to trust that you are connected to your higher power from within your Self.

Law 5: The Self must be nurtured to thrive.

The goal: Nurture your Self so that you can grow beyond your limiting beliefs and narratives.

Law 6: Unnurtured, the inner Self defaults to ingrained reactionary survival instincts.

The goal: Learn to see and interrupt your reactionary behavior.

Law 7: The inner Self is more powerful than external circumstances.

The goal: Discover the unseen and unengaged power within you.

These statements are factual. Use the 7 Laws of Self as tools to help you challenge the lies you carry about your Self. The next time you are feeling lost or down on your Self use one or all of the 7 Laws to help reframe your thinking: (1) I am made on purpose with a unique contribution; (2) I am enough; (3) remembering this is my power; (4) a higher power lives at the center of me; (5) daily, I must take time to remember and acknowledge the source of my life with gratitude; (6) when times are difficult, I must remember to meet the challenge, trusting that I never walk alone; (7) within me is endless strength, resilience, and wisdom that is more powerful than my circumstances. It is my responsibility to remember the truth and abide by the Laws that honor the inner Self.

It's time to look at how to take this journey now that we have established:

- The inner Self is different from the physical body—it supports wellbeing, whereas the physical body supports wellness; both are important.
- The Self comprises our thoughts, feelings, and beliefs, which drive our actions and reactions and impact our experience of life.
- The 7 Laws of Self are tools to help build a better relationship with the Self.

How to Take This Journey

READING THIS BOOK IS AN INTERACTIVE EXPERIENCE. YOU can engage with the 7 Laws of Self, the other tools and concepts, and the 14 Practices for Inner Health and Wellbeing immediately. Throughout your day, think about the concepts presented in this book, challenge them, and share your thoughts and experiences with others. Aim to engage with this content as an opportunity to spend quality time with your Self. If you already embrace a concept, see and experience it with fresh eyes and lead with an open, unbiased, and inquisitive mind. As you read, be curious and conscious about how to make the concepts actionable. Challenge the habit of thinking you already know yourself and spend time getting to know your Self.

At my Inner Fitness Workouts and events, I begin with two requests: First, have fun, and second, play full-out. This encourages participants to bring joy to investing in themselves—to consider and try the concepts in an open and curious way. Here are some other basic guidelines that will help you learn everything you need to know about becoming your whole Self as you begin to live it.

Curiosity and playfulness activate neural networks that encourage discovery and creativity, and enhance your ability to retain information. Playfulness also releases pleasure hormones that help reduce negative emotions and support a more positive and relaxed state of mind.

Talk to Your Self

Whenever you encounter the prompts "Say" or "Ask" in this book, speak **out loud** to yourself. Talking to yourself supports critical thinking and focus and signals to the brain that something is significant. Positive Self-talk can motivate, help reduce stress, and allow you to acknowledge and develop a relationship with your inner Self. And therein is the point of this journey—to engage, hang out with, and develop a relationship with your inner Self.

If emotions well up, acknowledge them; don't judge them. Say out loud: "I feel angry," or "I feel excited," or overwhelmed, sad, hopeful—whatever the case is for you. Acknowledging your emotions without judgment is vital to developing inner fitness.

Do the Exercises

Seize the opportunity. This book includes exercises that will allow you to spend reflective time with your Self. Engage with the exercises. This is how you practice inner fitness. The more you practice, the more connected to your Self you will become.

Take Your Time

Feel free to engage this book meditatively. Read a chapter or passage, and then let yourself mull over what resonates before you continue the journey. Every person's journey looks different, so give yourself permission to do what feels productive and helpful to you.

Use Your Heart and Gut

Listen to your heart and gut. Research says that the mind, heart, and gut are intelligent systems that communicate with one another, helping us make better decisions and have more profound insights. The gut holds information and activates our intuition, hence the term *gut instinct*. The heart has more neurons and energy than the brain. Notice when your heart resonates and opens, or resists and closes, and take note of the thoughts or feelings associated with your experience.

Understand the Difference Between Self and Selfish

In every workshop, someone confuses Self-care with selfishness or self-centeredness. The dictionary defines *selfishness* as lacking consideration for others and being chiefly concerned with personal profit or pleasure. Self-care, on the other hand, is the practice of taking an active role in protecting one's wellbeing and happiness, especially during periods of stress. This means learning to recognize and minimize the frequency of taking care of the needs of others at the expense of your mental and physical health and wellbeing. Most people who are worried about being selfish aren't in fact selfish. These people tend to be overly concerned with doing the right thing and taking care of others, often at a cost to themselves. However, these overextended people are selfless to a fault when it comes to taking care of themselves.

>> **EXERCISE: GRAB YOUR BASELINE**

You won't be the same at the end of this journey. In order to know how far your journey has brought you, you must know the point from where you begin—your baseline. Take a moment to rate where you are with your Self using the following eight statements. Before rating each statement, say aloud, "If I tell myself the truth . . ." Self-honesty is the fastest path to your whole Self. For the best experience on this journey, I highly recommend you complete this exercise before continuing.

On a scale of 1 to 10, 10 being the best it can possibly be and 1 being nonexistent, rate yourself regarding the following statements:

If I tell myself the truth . . .

1. I rate my belief in myself at _____.
2. I rate my personal thriving at _____.
3. I rate being controlled by limiting beliefs at _____.
4. I rate feeling capable at _____.
5. I rate feeling controlled by old patterns or issues at _____.
6. I rate feeling stuck in an important area of my life at _____.
7. I rate feeling not good enough at _____ or not smart enough at _____.
8. I rate my desire to change my life for the better at _____.

The first seven assessment statements help you objectively see the landscape of your relationship with your inner Self. The last statement is the most important. Your desire to change drives everything. If you desire change, change will happen.

Engage with Random Stories

Throughout this book, I've included what I call "Not-So-Random Stories" illustrating the internal work of inner fitness and varied perspectives. Though the stories are "random," be open to seeing how the story might relate to your life.

Set an Intention to Become the Person You Want to Be

Many people set goals focused on the physical things they want: marriage, a career, a promotion, or a house. Fewer people focus on who they want to be and how they want to feel inside. I dated a brilliant guy who achieved extraordinary success in the world. However, he lamented his lack of loyalty and integrity. It never occurred to him that he could also focus on becoming more loyal and having impeccable integrity.

Inner fitness requires considering the person you want to be and how you want to feel internally, and adopting behaviors that support your intention.

Intentions and goals are two sides of the same coin. An intention is the inner state you want to achieve; goals are the individual objectives or roadmap for getting there. My intention was to live a life that was fit for my soul. A few of my goals for getting there were to become an actress, continually grow as a person, and always live below my financial means to mitigate stress from the unsteady income of an actor.

When you set intentions, you're cultivating the mindset, heartset, and energy necessary to evolve into a whole version of yourself day-by-day. Over the years I have rewritten and edited my intentions and goals. The following is the intention statement I now share at workshops and conferences. The following intention statement invites you to be curious, courageous, and compassionate with yourself as you work toward living well and thriving. These intentions help you step into the role of the author of your life story and live each day as an opportunity to practice living in alignment with your inner Self.

I encourage you to say this intention out loud.

Live Well and Thrive

INTENTION STATEMENT

I AIM TO LIVE WELL AND THRIVE!

I SET THE INTENTION

—TO GET COURAGEOUSLY CURIOUS ABOUT MY LIFE!

—TO SEE WHAT NEEDS TO BE SEEN IN MY LIFE!

I AIM TO LIVE WELL AND THRIVE!

I SET THE INTENTION

—TO HEAL WHAT NEEDS TO BE HEALED IN MY LIFE!

—TO STAND INSIDE MYSELF WITH MY ARMS STRETCHED WIDE!

—TO TURN AROUND 360 DEGREES AND NOT BUMP INTO ANY

YOU-KNOW-WHAT!

I AIM TO LIVE WELL AND THRIVE!

I SET THE INTENTION

—TO HAVE FUN!

—TO SHINE!

—TO SHOW UP FOR MYSELF AND MY LIFE 1,000 PERCENT!

I AIM TO LIVE WELL AND THRIVE!

AND TO LOVE MYSELF SO MUCH

THAT I CAN LOVE YOU!

I aim to live well and thrive!

What is your intention for your life, and what are three goals that will help you get there? According to a study conducted by psychology professor Gail Matthews regarding goal-setting, if we take the extra step of writing our goals down, we are much more likely to achieve them.

>> EXERCISE: SET YOUR INTENTION

Write down your intention for how you want to be and feel
inside and three goals:

My intention for my inner Self is _____.

Three goals that support my intention:

1. _____.

2. _____.

3. _____.

Sample exercise:

My intention for my inner Self is _greater freedom and joy_ .

Three goals that support my intention:

1. _Work with a therapist_ .

2. _Do things that expand my comfort zone_ .

3. _Develop friendships with positive people_ .

It follows that when you apply intention-setting to developing
your inner Self and write down how you want to feel and respond
to life, you are much more likely to become who you want to be and
feel how you want to feel.

Writing down your intention or goal is the first time it becomes tangible; you can pick up your journal and touch and read
the words. The physical effort of writing down your goals and intentions, whether on paper or a device, breathes life into what is
otherwise a potentially fleeting thought. Your goal or dream now
"lives" in the physical world in a way you can hold and refer to. This
holding place acts as a magnet, drawing you and your goals together
and helping to fulfill your intention.

Investing time and effort into clarifying your thoughts and
working with them is an example of giving your Self attention.

Adopt the intention statement "Live Well and Thrive" if it resonates with you, or go to our resource page at TheInnerFitnessProject .com, print it, and tailor it to yourself. Don't stress over getting your intention statement perfect. Your life is a work in progress, and so is your intention for your life. You can tweak and refine it as often as you like. You can even create a daily intention to help you remember how you want to think and respond each day or how you relate to a specific challenge or event. Spending five or ten minutes with your Self, first thing in the morning or before you go to bed, will help you practice honoring your Self.

Use the following template to help you stay connected to your inner Self:

>> **EXERCISE: YOUR DAILY INTENTION**

Set an intention for how you want to be in a relationship with your inner Self. Example: *I set the intention to discover and value my Self.* Let your intention flow from your heart. Your intention's length is up to you.

My intention for my Self today is _____.

I want to be better at _____.

I want to be aware of _____.

I want to let go of _____.

I want to trust _____.

A Not-So-Random Story About Intention

I learned the power of setting an intention at twenty-six years old when I attended an all-day real estate course that I found in a weekly throwaway paper. At the time, I knew nothing about real estate, but I had read *Rich Dad Poor Dad* by Robert T. Kiyosaki. In the book, he says that real estate is a proven way that the average person can build wealth. In that course, I learned about probate sales.

Probate is the process a deceased person's assets go through when they die without a will. The court steps in, sells those assets, and pays any outstanding financial obligations. A probate property sale often starts at a price below market value. This makes the right property a great opportunity. Plus, at least back then, first-time buyers had the advantage of paying only 5 percent down. One of my goals toward achieving my intention to become a working actress was to have income property.

I set the intention: Find a probate property.

Within eighteen months of taking that real estate class, with zero savings and living in a five-hundred-square-foot studio apartment, I found myself the owner of a little craftsman house on Thirtieth Street in the Adams District of Los Angeles. Here's how that happened:

Out of the blue, my then-boss offered to loan me $3,500 to buy a new car to replace my beat-up Volkswagen fastback that was often in the auto repair shop. She offered that I could repay her monthly out of my paycheck. I asked her whether she would still loan me the money if I used it to buy a house instead of a car. She laughed and said, "Sure, I will loan you the money if you can buy a house for $3,500." I found a probate property, went into a bidding war with Realtors, and walked out of court with my first house. I paid just $50,000 for it with a 5 percent down payment, with closing costs borrowed from my parents and friends.

I never lived in that first house. I couldn't afford to! Instead, I rented it out and made enough money to pay my boss back quicker than planned. I sold that little house three years later, moved out of the studio apartment that had been my home for ten years, and into a duplex I purchased on the south end of the Wilshire District in Los Angeles.

Owning that first house fulfilled the goal of the financial freedom I needed to build my acting career. I was convinced that setting that intention and having that goal positively affected me. So I began to lead with a clear intention in every important area of my life.

Setting an intention with and for yourself puts you in an active relationship with the vision you desire for your life and helps you remember your vision when life overwhelms or distracts you.

Okay. Let's begin the journey!

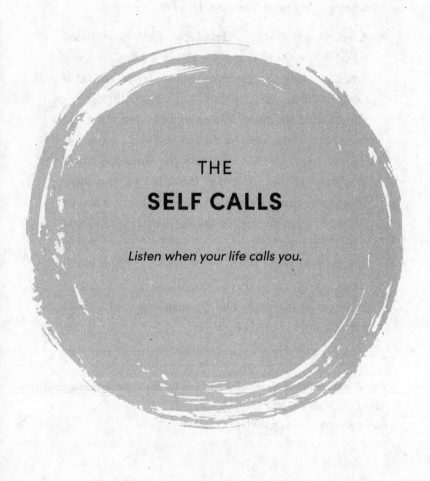

THE
SELF CALLS

Listen when your life calls you.

A Fairy Tale About Reconnecting with Your Self

A weary traveler sat by a calm lake, too tired to swim. They closed their eyes and daydreamed about the water washing over their body, clearing away sadness, regret, and other forms of fatigue, Self-rejection, and neglect. Then something tickled their skin. Their eyes flew open. They had thought they were alone on the secluded bank, but a smiling face was in the water. Startled, the weary one turned around to see who stood over them. No one was there. They slowly turned their head back to the lake just in time to catch the smiling face in the water turning to look at them. There was something vaguely familiar, yet mostly forgotten about the face in the water—something worth remembering. The weary one looked into the familiar eyes of the person moving toward the open water and, without warning, dove in to be saved.

A part of you remembers that you are whole, unbreakable, and full of possibilities. It holds you close and tight, awaiting the moment you can hold its truth for yourself.

Saying "Yes" to Your Self

————

YOU WOULDN'T PICK UP A BOOK ABOUT DISCOVERING YOUR Self without first knowing or sensing there is a Self waiting for you to either connect or reconnect with it. We all know there is more to us than the small, fearful, and less authentic person living our lives. Probably, you have felt "something" is missing from your life without being able to put your finger on it and call it by name. Maybe you hope this book can help you find it. You are not alone.

We all feel there is more to us than the life we currently know. This isn't wishful thinking; it is intuition. Our futures call us. Our unlived dreams and possibilities poke at us and cause us to reach for more. This is how we grow and move beyond our smaller ideas of ourselves.

The nature of the universe is to constantly grow and expand. Science tells us the universe began as a tiny pinprick that continues to expand and reveal its infinite nature; this is our nature, too. You and I have within us endless space and capacity to unfold into more of who we are. A part of us knows this. This is why watching the sunset at the beach or staring at the sky is so satisfying; it reminds us that we can experience the physical world with greater inner freedom, peace, and awe. Cultivating our inner fitness helps us expand and experience more of ourselves.

Say:

I feel there is more to me, and I desire to discover more of who I am.

Without a strong connection to our inner Self, we can drift away from a healthy sense of what is possible for our lives and the ability to be honest with ourselves, and end up living a life that is inauthentic. It takes a Self to say "no" to the parts of life we do not want and "yes" to the parts we do. It takes a Self to know our desires and to love ourselves and others.

When I share inner fitness work with people online or in a workshop, I ask them to check in with themselves and share why they are saying "yes" to their Selves and why they would like to begin the inner fitness journey. Here are some responses:

- I got lost doing everything for everybody else.
- I was trying to fulfill all the needs and expectations of everyone in my life.
- I was taught to just suck it up and keep pushing.
- I am rich. I'm supposed to be happy. But I'm not.
- I keep trying to be perfect, and the more I try, the more unhappy I become.
- I felt like everything in my life controlled me.
- I compromised my idea of love and happiness and settled for less.
- I have trust issues that I didn't even know I have.
- I lead, fix, rescue, and have answers for everyone except myself.
- I didn't realize there was more to me than my ability to provide.
- I was once myself, but life took me in a different direction and I lost myself.

- I used to be joyous, but now I'm an evil, angry person all the time.
- I always have to be together and strong, and the façade is too much.
- I have stress at work and in my personal life, and it's just too much.
- I know there is a part of me that I should have been paying attention to.

In the same way that a healthier physical body awaits underneath our bad eating habits, weight, flabby muscles, and lack of sleep, a more fulfilled and resilient Self awaits underneath our habitual worries, doubts, fears, harsh Self-judgment, limiting beliefs, and unconscious behavior.

So we must adopt strategies and practices that foster connection. When the light of our authentic Self becomes dimmed, distorted, or obliterated for any reason, we become less connected to our Self. No matter how successful or together we appear to the external world, inwardly, we carry the burden of our loss of Self. Inner fitness acknowledges that ongoing inner repair and strengthening are necessary to live life with strong and rewarding inner wellbeing. Awakening to our disconnection from Self is the first step toward discovering our whole Self.

>> EXERCISE: CHECK IN

Checking in with your Self is like chatting with a loved and trusted friend who acknowledges and affirms your inner Self. Take a moment to check in with your Self and state why you are taking this journey.

I have felt _____. I sense there is more to my life. I want _____.

My Return to Self

Your life is the closest thing to you. Listen to it.

I HAD BEEN PROGRESSING IN MY RELATIONSHIP WITH MY Self for two decades. Then one day, everything inside sped up, and thoughts that had gnawed at me for some time took center stage.

One morning while washing dishes in the early 2000s, "something" told me to search the Bible for the word *self*. The urge to search the Bible was unusual. Although I went to Sunday school every week for years when I was growing up, I don't consider myself a religious person. But I am a *spiritual* person, and during the building of my spiritual foundation, I attended the Agape Spiritual Center twice a week from 1986 to 1996.

That morning, I turned the kitchen faucet off and headed to my office. Seated at my big clunky computer, I typed "biblical concordance" into the search engine. In a random concordance search bar, I typed the word *self*. Nothing came up.

Thinking I had done something wrong, I typed *self* again. Nothing again. I thought, *How can this be? The word* self *must be in the Bible.*

I typed and hit enter a third time and got the same results.

Was there really no mention of *self* in the Bible?

For weeks, I ruminated on the absence of the word *self* in one of the most revered human stories and texts. I pondered with friends the possible impact the absence of *self* in the Bible could have on our collective psyche. Don't we matter? Could the lack of valuing ourselves be why people are so harsh with themselves? We are taught to be kind to others, but what about being kind to ourselves? Was this how we've come to give so much to others and leave ourselves out of our lives?

The absence of *self* disturbed me. For the first time, I stopped and deliberately contemplated the importance of this four-letter word. The inner Self instigates our thoughts, molds our feelings, drives our choices, and governs our sense of what's possible. A vague thought sharpened: Society is slow to acknowledge the inner Self and its needs. Historically, our inner world largely goes unexplored and unchallenged as though it is inconsequential. We acknowledge and even glorify the physical body. But our thoughts, feelings, and beliefs, and the actions and reactions they drive, are not viewed as directly related to our experience of life. **As we begin to see our thoughts, feelings, and beliefs as the building blocks of our experiences, we learn to turn them into tools and create our lives more intentionally.**

It felt absurd that something so fundamental to our existence as Self could be minimized, misunderstood, underaddressed, and taken for granted. I yearned for internal personal power, but I didn't know how to achieve it. How are we to "know thyself," as great thinkers advise, when mention of the Self is avoided or viewed as self-centered and therefore taboo?

If we don't have a healthy relationship with our Self, we are screwed. We are left with feeling inadequate or not good enough, tortured by our minds and the idea that everyone else has it together while we flail trying to figure life out. Without insight into our thoughts, fears, and beliefs, how can we hope for inner comfort or peace or navigate to our dreams? For myself, how would I over-come my stage fright and have the career of my dreams?

As a result of my inner turmoil, I became more curious about the Self that was inside my body yet was so much more than my physical body.

Say:
The way to reconnect with my Self is to acknowledge its existence and spend time getting to know my Self.

What Happens When Our Joy Is Attacked

Growing up, I often heard an adult (not my parents, thankfully) say, "Go sit your fast-ass down." (Depending on your culture, you might relate to a different version of this admonishment, but you get my point.) This was a reprimand a child received for doing something clever, smart, or unexpected, or acting older or wiser than their age. In other words, a child's gifts or uniqueness could attract adult dis-pleasure and management of that child's behavior or very being.

A negative response to another's joy or excitement has turned many joyous moments into shameful, self-conscious ones. Such sour responses to a child's joy cause that child to feel less confident about who they are and what parts of themselves are acceptable. This kind of emotional stress teaches the child, bit by bit, to be-come less authentic and to need another's approval to feel whole. The Canadian-Hungarian physician and author Gabor Maté says that if a child receives the message from a caregiver that they are unacceptable as they are, the child often will adapt and reshape themselves to be perceived as acceptable by the people responsible for their survival needs.

When a healthy focus on Self is met with judgment, dismissal, or disdain, we are being taught that expressing ourselves or being proud of ourselves or our achievements is wrong. We learn that respect for Self is the same as thinking we are better than another. Such reactions to our Self are not cautionary wisdom. They reject the divinity within the Self. Over time, such rejection leads to a disconnection from our Self. The current lack of Self-care in our families and the world and the damage it is causing make this misconceived mindset dangerous.

Everyone Deserves Permission to Shine

We should want young people—heck, everyone—to be able to stand in front of a mirror and appreciate the image they see and to feel like they walk with power inside them. Then, every person could feel good, capable, and full of Self, with respectful Self-consideration, inner resilience, and the strength to grow beyond stifling experiences. If the universe is aware of us—as seems to be the case because of a connection between what we think and what manifests in our lives (I say more about this below)—then that awareness must cause us to pause and question our choices or feel supported in our decisions. We can all be encouraged to add to the world the unique gifts that are tied to our fingerprints.

Self Is Not a Negative Term

I was obsessed with the disconnect from and unwarranted disrespect of the Self. The need to champion Self felt imperative. I began to take the grammatical license to separate and capitalize the word *Self* whenever it felt appropriate, as a reminder to myself to honor my inner Self. I ruminated on why the Self is automatically associated with characteristics that need to be rejected, managed, or disowned. Selfishness, self-centeredness, arrogance, egotistical conceit, or narcissism do not accurately represent nor support the whole Self. They undermine. I wondered aloud how we all could spend more time with thoughts, feelings, beliefs, actions, and reactions that could make our lives better.

If hurt people hurt other people, then it seemed to me that people who practice Self-respect and Self-love are more likely to treat others with respect and care. In *The Myth of Normal: Trauma, Illness, and Healing in a Toxic Culture*, Gabor Maté proffers the possibility that behind every unloving or hurtful act committed by an individual is a Self that was treated poorly, rejected, or ignored and longs to be reunited with the joy, peace, and Self-trust they had before trauma changed their life.

A healthy, loving relationship with our Self is our best hope for living a joyous life despite the difficult life events we have encountered, such as poor parenting, lack of education, abuse, and trauma. I couldn't stop thinking about how we can rethink and redesign our relationship with Self. A bit of a riddle began to form: How do I see the Self that hides in plain sight?

Listen to Your Intuitive Self

One day while I was driving, an inner nudge said, *Go to the Bodhi Tree Bookstore.* Out loud, to thin air, I asked, "Why?" Then I obediently headed to the bookstore that had been famous since the 1970s. Looking back, I was learning to listen to my Self.

A rare parking spot in front of the store was waiting for me. I moved into the crowded store wondering what I was supposed to do next. I have had numerous moments that felt guided and divine, but nothing quite like that one. With little hesitation, in a bookstore filled with spiritual books of all kinds, dealing with every belief system and culture in the world, I was drawn to a room in the back of the store that, in all my years shopping at the Bodhi Tree, I had never ventured into before. But that day, I was guided to enter it. I stood there for a few beats, staring at the shelving that went almost to the ceiling on three and a half walls, with two or three metal racks in the center, all filled with books. I exhaled and said out loud, "Now what?"

I slowly walked around one of the center bookshelves. Then, one lone book fell off the shelf onto the floor. The title was *Be As You Are: The Teachings of Sri Ramana Maharshi*, an Indian Hindu sage whom I had never heard of.

I opened the book.

It was about the Self.

It addressed the questions that most occupied my mind and heart at the time.

How could I reduce such a tailor-made experience to coincidence? I felt like I was *seen*, and that I mattered to an unseen force. This is the power that comes with having a clear and resonating intention.

I read the book from cover to cover in a day or two. Then I read it again.

In terms of the Self, I discovered: *You are the thing you are searching for.* I was left with the very clear realization that we all can make our lives better by honoring ourselves—giving the Self quality time, feeding our minds with information that heals and interrupts our hurtful stories, and learning to *understand* instead of judging the Self amid adversity.

Reprogram Your Thoughts

Reclaiming our whole Self requires seeing and rewiring the deeply ingrained and subtle habits of Self-judgment, Self-attack, and Self-rejection. Instead, we must practice addressing the Self with respect, understanding, and compassion.

Say:

I deserve my respect, understanding, and compassion.

Often, when I'm speaking before an audience, someone voices concern that focusing on Self undermines family and community. My response: When we see our Self as an expression of our higher power, then respect of Self is far from indulgent. It makes us responsible for our actions and choices—which in turn enhances family and community.

Discovery of Self is every person's encoded purpose. It is the fastest path to experiencing our connection to a higher power. Like the acorn's purpose is to grow into an oak tree, living as our whole Self—knowing why we do what we do, understanding and honoring feelings, navigating life purposefully, actively reclaiming Self from hurtful experiences, and discovering our innate worthiness—is how we become human versions of a strong, resilient, bold, and beautiful oak tree.

There are many lessons to be learned in this life. One of the most surprising is that how we feel about ourselves feeds our joy and sorrow. Therefore, learning to see and attend to the Self is crucial.

Say:
When I love and honor my Self, I acknowledge and honor
the intelligent force that created me, and I become known to
myself.

Want More

You might wonder how I acquired such an active relationship with my Self.

I wanted it.

Even before I understood what a relationship with Self might entail, I wanted something more within myself. Wanting more of anything—Self, freedom from our challenges, understanding, hope, joy—is a necessary step to obtaining it. Global spiritual leader and

Buddhist monk Thich Nhat Hanh explained that it is impossible to have a "right" side without having a left. The right cannot be pulled or separated from the left. Cut the left side off, and another left takes its place. One creates the other. This makes the right and left one, not two.

Within our desire for freedom is a lack of freedom that makes the idea of freedom possible. As Thich Nhat Hanh famously said, *No mud, no lotus.*

Say:
In my mud is a beautiful flower.

In Every Change Profound Inner Growth Awaits

I took Thich Nhat Hanh's "no right without a left" analogy to heart and applied it to all dualities—good/bad, conscious/unconscious, up/down. The two sides were inextricably connected. My elementary school stage fright hell meant great freedom was also present. I realized that my difficulty offered me a gift as big as the problem. The difficulty was the "mud" necessary to birth the "flower" of wisdom and a deeper understanding of my Self. This aha moment changed how I encountered all challenges and eventually led to my passion for inner fitness, and later to my creating the Inner Fitness Project, and now to my sharing the details of such discoveries in this book.

These are examples of the profound discoveries that were part of my difficult journey. But gaining the "flowers" required skillfully working with the problem. I went looking for answers and endeavored to turn whatever information I found into action, no matter how unsophisticated my attempt.

Working with my Self, with the expectation of expanding, stretched my sense of Self and capacity to be with life more courageously and effectively. I leaned into the idea that the mud was evidence that something beautiful was being created. I saw that all creations are preceded by a journey that usually involves pain or effort. This thinking changed how I perceived and related to all internal dis-ease. I turned internal freedom into a destination, and problems and emotional difficulties into a path to greater freedom.

Ask:

What beauty is being created by the mud in my life?

 A Tool: EEQs

The question *What beauty is being created by the mud in my life?* is what I call an effective and empowering question (or EEQ). Asking an EEQ is a tool that adjusts your orientation to an issue or problem. If fear, overwhelm, or doubt is present, asking an EEQ makes room for you to address the situation with curiosity instead of running from it.

EEQs are *how, what, who,* or *where* questions that create mental, emotional, and spiritual openness and unlock the subconscious mind so that answers or next steps can emerge. (Avoid *why* questions because they keep you stuck in the problem versus leading you to answers or solutions; I discuss this more in Practice 2 and below.)

This openness is the setup for turning the problem before you into a life-enhancing opportunity. An EEQ is *effective* because any answer to the question moves you in the direction you desire. Any answer to the question *What beauty is being created by the mud in my life?* will move you toward beauty or benefit. The question is *empowering* because it reframes how you see a difficulty and opens your eyes to a positive outcome.

Get Curious

The subconscious remembers and stores everything, all the thoughts and feelings we've ever experienced; it knows and is sensitive to our shared human experiences. Within the subconscious is wisdom about life, death, and living aligned with your Self.

Being curious about and looking for answers invites answers into our lives.

If we see ourselves as extensions of a universal force, then we can imagine our minds as connected to the intelligence of the universe. Asking the universe an open-ended question is like typing a question into the best search engine, which immediately finds answers that "match" the question.

For example, if you ask the question "Why does this always happen to me?" the answers might be things like "Because you don't follow through," "Because you lead with insecurity and make poor choices," "Because you lack trust." **(Check your heart and stomach right now and see how reading these answers makes you feel.)** Answers to *why* questions don't empower. They feel awful and keep you stuck in the problem and can even make the problem feel bigger or insurmountable. They waste time. It is like the old saying "You can't plant apples and expect to get oranges." You asked *why*, so in an "apples-to-apples" way, the answer will match the *why* question.

Asking a *how*, *what*, *who*, or *where* question is a more direct route to getting answers that move you forward. For instance, if you ask "How can I achieve the results I desire?" the answer will reveal things you can do, steps you can take, or insights that help you move forward.

Designing questions in such a way that the answers effectively fulfill the question is the key to creating effective and empowering questions. EEQs keep you open and available to answers and possibilities beyond what you know or can see. An EEQ is the perfect way to proceed in life when you are struck and you don't know which way to go. (I talk more about EEQs in Practice 2.)

My Skill-Building Practice

While driving, sitting alone, or writing in my journal, I would ask questions out loud:

- *What must I know or see to deepen my sense of Self?*
- *How can I respond in a way that supports my growth and empowers my decision-making, healing, or understanding of my Self and life?*
- *How can I know greater internal freedom?*

Each question represented my giving quality time and consideration to my Self and inviting in the idea of being in partnership with an unseen force.

I held EEQs inside me throughout my day like they were a meditation or prayer—always in the background, talking to my subconscious. They helped me practice being with uncomfortable feelings and events without judging myself: I learned to allow myself to feel discomfort without creating a negative story. Instead of saying *This thing happened to me and I feel like a victim*, the narrative became merely *This thing happened.*

Life was bumping into life, creating more life.

Asking a good question, where the aim was simply to ask the question without expecting an answer two minutes later, taught me patience and to be in an active relationship with my Self and the universe. I realized that if I was actively looking for freedom, a part of me was not in bondage. There was more to me than the habit of feeling at the mercy of a problem.

A Tool: Creating More Life

Life Is Bumping into Life, Creating More Life. This is a simple visualization and mindset that can help us navigate life's difficulties and chaos without taking it personally. The nature of the universe is creative. We humans, too, are creative by nature. When the creativity of the universe bumps into our creative nature, how we respond creates something—an emotional mood that impacts how we respond, and how we respond impacts what happens next.

Developing the habit of responding with the mindset that *life is bumping into life, creating more life*—that is, *don't take it personally*—is a wise way of moving forward and making conscious choices rather than taking life personally and becoming a victim of circumstances. When we don't take life personally, we sidestep the compulsion to create a negative or hurtful narrative, and we are free to address any issue or need more objectively and with a level head. Seeing circumstances through this lens allows us to acknowledge the circumstances and move on.

As you go through your day, if, for instance, a person cuts you off in traffic or a person you were expecting to meet doesn't show up, or anything else displeasing occurs, to put it in a healthy perspective, say out loud: **"Life is bumping into life, creating more life."** Don't take it personally and move on.

By constructively hanging out with myself—(1) asking open-ended questions, (2) expending **EFFORT** (Extracting Freedom

From Our Restricted Thinking), and (3) challenging my limited understanding of myself—I was taking practical steps toward a deeper, more secure relationship with the Self. I dared to trust that my sincere contemplation of my Self was as meaningful as the effort that mystics or spiritual gurus exert. Anyone wanting to experience themselves more deeply can do the same.

Ask:
How can I create a life that is a perfect fit for me?

Takeaways:
- You have an inner Self that matters.
- Be curious, listen, and attend to your Self.
- Want more; ask effective and empowering questions.

>> EXERCISE: CREATE THE RELATIONSHIP YOU WANT WITH YOUR SELF

Identify an area of challenge in your life and imagine the kind of relationship you want to have with your Self regarding this challenge.

Example: *Area of challenge*—In meetings I become hyper self-conscious and critical of myself. *Relationship I want with my Self*—I want to feel free and capable in meetings, and so prepared and ready to share that I forget about being self-conscious and words flow from me clearly and effectively. I want people to comment on how great my presentations are.

Taking time to imagine and commit to paper, or on your device, how you want to experience your Self in your areas of challenge is a perfect way to mine good from difficulty and create the life you want.

A Tool: Up Until Now

Up Until Now, and From This Point Forward. This elegant tool allows you to honestly acknowledge where you are in your life and gives you the green light to move beyond where you are. It is perfect for shifting your thinking toward possibilities and away from feeling stuck or trapped by how things have historically been. Here's how it works: *Up until now*, life has been however it's been, but *from this point forward*, things can change for the better. I encourage you to take a moment and say the phrase again, aloud: *Up until now*, life has been however it's been, but *from this point forward*, things can change for the better. Did you feel an opening occur inside you? This phrase creates a sense of possibility based upon an irrefutable truth: Things in your life can always change for the better. Science confirms this. The brain can change throughout your entire life, up to the very end. This means you are never stuck and you don't have to feel handcuffed to your past or old behavior or unhelpful emotions or ways of thinking. From this point forward, things can change for the better. This tool helps you remember that greater freedom, joy, peace, and love are possible. Use the tool often. Allow it to reset your thinking, encourage your progress, and help you boldly say "no" to things or ways of responding that you no longer want to engage with. This is how we can use this pair of phrases to transform our lives: When you are talking to yourself or others and you catch yourself taking the same old stance, holding the same old beliefs, or seeing in the same old ways, stop. Rethink and restate using *up until now, and from this point forward*.

>> EXERCISE: UP UNTIL NOW AND FROM THIS POINT FORWARD

Take a moment and identify at least two scenarios that you can apply *Up until now, and from this point forward* to. Use the sentence prompt below to help guide you.

Up until now __(state your old issue or behavior)__, but from this point forward, it can change for the better.

These uncommon prompts and tools build inner fitness. Applying them in your daily navigation of life is revolutionary.

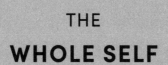

THE
WHOLE SELF

To see your whole Self look beyond what you see.

The Dream of Self

JUST AS I WAS BEGINNING TO SEE AND REVERE THE SELF, I had a dream in 2008 that changed my understanding of the Self and provided the *Three Selves framework* that helped define my inner fitness journey and can be helpful to you, too. Here's my Dream of Self:

A curious woman walked along a secluded, overcast beach, dreaming of her life and enjoying the sand beneath her feet. Up ahead she saw two women arguing. Not wanting to intrude, the Dreamer turned to go back in the opposite direction, but to her surprise, her feet continued moving closer to the arguing pair.

As she approached them, it became clear that only one of the two women was arguing. The one with her back to the ocean was flailing her arms and stomping her feet. But the other woman, facing the arguing one and the ocean, stood quietly—no fight in her at all. The arguing woman noticed the Dreamer coming toward them and became louder and more animated. But the Dreamer could not hear the shouting voice, for the sight of the quiet calm of the compelling woman held her attention.

The Dreamer stopped just ten feet away from the pair. The argumentative woman's eyes were filled with angry words that were never spoken because, without warning, the compelling one, with all her stillness, glanced at the Dreamer, then stepped forward and wrapped her arms around the arguing one, drew her in, and held her close. The arguing woman resisted at first, out of habit. But as her habit of fear and resistance melted, the arguing woman went limp and rested in the other's arms—the love settling her fight.

The Dreamer wondered, *Who are these women?* Then, the embracing pair turned toward the Dreamer, who stared back at them in disbelief—for the Dreamer's face belonged to all three. The curious woman—the Dreamer—joined the embrace. And arm in arm the three of them—*the surviving self, the thriving Self, and the infinite SELF*—walked the beach in harmony.

(You can visit YouTube and search for "@tinalifford dream" and watch the five minute and thirty-one second film that depicts my dream.)

Say:
We are all more than we know or give ourselves credit for being.

I don't dream often. When I do, I rarely remember my dreams. But the Dream of Self was more than just a dream. It was an answer to a heart-held desire to know and understand my Self and become comfortable with every aspect of my inner Self. The dream became my teacher. To this day I continue to turn to it for guidance.

The Three Selves

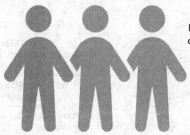

Surviving self fears there's something wrong and looks for it.

Infinite SELF accepts and affirms life as it is.

Thriving Self embraces the good and growth in everything and looks for it.

WHAT IF THE SELF THAT SITS IN YOUR SEAT RIGHT NOW is not one self (as you have come to know yourself) but three selves? One is focused on surviving, another on thriving, and the third is an infinite SELF that is the intelligent force behind life.

What if these selves form the whole inner Self, with a range of distinct, identifiable characteristics that influence and dictate all your behavior?

The notion of a range to our psyches is not new. Sigmund Freud's id, ego, and superego; Abraham Maslow's hierarchy of needs; Christianity's holy trinity; and even the theory of the brain's triune structure—the reptilian brain, the paleomammalian brain (limbic system), and the neomammalian brain (neocortex)—speak of a range of psychological characteristics and associated behaviors.

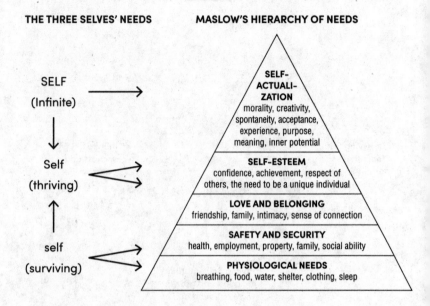

But my Dream of Self gave me a simple, relatable view of my Self. We all have experienced moments of depression, joy, and profound wisdom. I could see the range of Self within me that worries and fears, that hopes and dreams, and that is intuitive and wise. This range had been there all the time, but in the dream, I saw I could turn to this view of my Self to better understand and manage my internal world.

The Three Selves framework of the surviving self, the thriving Self, and the infinite SELF describes internal experiences we all know. This range of Self lives in each of us and, when balanced, makes the whole Self. However, there are no hard lines that define these Three Selves, no clear point where one "self" ends and the other begins. Like water that gathers itself into a wave and then relaxes as it rolls up the beach, we move in and out of the Three Selves countless times throughout every day. Something triggers fear or self-doubt, and our panic or uncertainty calls forth the surviving self. Grabbing hold of a compelling idea or dream and feeling recharged with hope or expanding our sense of possibility and acting courageously is the thriving Self. Having an inner knowing that ushers in profound understanding, acceptance, and peace is the infinite SELF.

To see the Self in action and experience its full range, we must know what to look for and then look often to see which mindset, or which "Self," drives our thoughts, feelings, beliefs, actions, and reactions.

The Surviving Self

The surviving self is the arguing self that is always ready for a fight, takes life personally, lacks the ability to manage its reactive nature, and leads with worry, doubt, and fear. This self focuses on survival above all else and constantly sees itself at risk. It attacks first in fear of being attacked and is always defending and proving itself. Our fight for survival can be physical or financial, can be based in beliefs, can be about our reputation or how we see ourselves or prefer to be seen, and is mostly unconscious.

The surviving self is terrified that something devastating will happen that we won't be able to manage. Governed by the "reptilian brain," the oldest part of the brain, the surviving self defaults to worry, doubt, and fear; looks for threats or danger; and operates from the fight, flight, or freeze response. This self is quick to judge itself and others and is so consumed with survival that it is not aware of the higher ranges within it.

The mindset of the surviving self is: *Something's wrong and against me; so watch out!*

SEEING MY SURVIVING SELF

Before my Dream of Self, I did not see how often I operated from the surviving self. I hadn't heard the term *surviving self* until it came to me to describe the realizations offered in the dream. I wasn't aware of what it meant to be in survival mode. I didn't know what to look for or the feelings that represent and drive the surviving self. I avoided my feelings to distance myself from emotional discomfort, insecurity, and a sense of loss or fear. I viewed feelings as a hindrance to the push-forward, go-get-'em messaging of human potential gurus. I distracted myself from my feelings with busyness.

I hadn't yet learned that feelings support us in being our whole Self and play a crucial role in mental health. They provide warning signs when we are at risk of denying our truth, compromising our integrity, or disowning parts of ourselves. And they support healthy, honest communication with others and the ability to trust oneself and foster resilience. Acknowledging, exploring, or honoring our feelings helps us process events in real time as opposed to avoiding feelings and ignoring discomfort or hurt. The more we avoid our feelings instead of understanding them or allow unaddressed hurt to course through our nervous systems, the more disconnected from our Self we become.

In my Dream of Self, the surviving self was using flailing arms, stomping feet, and pounding fists to communicate. This part of us always looks for what's wrong or is at war with something and needs to prove itself or its value. Unconsciously, it constantly brings its hurtful past into the present, keeping the past hurt an active memory and continuing source of pain.

We all have reacted poorly in new situations where an unhealed pain from the past was triggered.

I set the intention to sit in my observer's chair and catch sight of my surviving self behavior.

A Tool: The Observer's Chair

The observer's chair is a tool you can use to identify and see unconscious behavior. Imagine that you are sitting above your life watching it like a movie. This objectivity allows you to see yourself in action and widens your ability to view events and circumstances from a different perspective. When you watch a movie, you know and see things that the characters in the movie cannot.

It wasn't easy for me to see how often I was at war with life because I tend to be composed until I'm not. (When I'm not, I can go from zero to a hundred in seconds.) Because I'm easygoing and not prone to obvious tantrums, I had to be intentional and look beyond my composed physicality to the energy inside me to catch sight of my surviving self.

But from my observer's chair, I clearly saw the surviving self.

Often, I was irritated, dismissive, and judgmental, and fought to be right. I would disagree and assume I was right without leaving room for the possibility that other people were as creative, smart, and capable as me. If I'm honest with myself, seeing these truths wasn't shocking.

There was plenty of evidence that this energy lived in me. A part of me was aware of when I was leading with this telltale behavior. I just had not taken the time to explore and own it. My surviving self mindset was as present to me, yet unacknowledged by me, as water is to a fish. Why fix what feels natural and right? Thoughts that move us to defend ourselves and judge others are appropriate and reasonable thoughts for the surviving self, who lives life comparing, judging, and othering—habitually seeing through the lens of something being wrong and being at odds with something or someone.

I began to curate a list of surviving self characteristics that could help me pause and question my thoughts and behavior to determine whether I was appropriately or unconsciously operating in survival mode. The words on the surviving self word graphic below are some of the more common ones that signal we are operating from our surviving self.

>> EXERCISE: YOUR SURVIVING SELF HABITS

Against-Me Thinking   Anger   Guilt   Blame

Aggression   Assumptions   Depression

Despair   Jealousy   Doubt   Fear   Isolation

surviving self | The surviving self represents the part of us that reacts to life. Quick to judge and take things personally, the surviving self is always ready for a fight.

War   Judgment   Oppression   Shame   Worry

Lack   Hatred   Powerlessness   Victimization

Negativity   Revenge   Rage

Without judging your Self, circle in the word graphic (or create a list of) your three most common surviving self habits.

OTHER SURVIVING SELF SIGHTINGS

In my surviving self workshop, people share ways their surviving self shows up in their lives. Some of them might seem familiar to you:

- When things get difficult or challenging, I go numb and unconsciously revert to the habits of my surviving self.
- I resort to protecting myself and blaming others; I see enemies everywhere and justify attacking them before they can attack me.
- I see myself being a person I don't want to be, but I can't seem to interrupt the habit.
- I get stuck replaying the past.
- I get angry because of things that happened in my life and feel justified in treating other people poorly.
- I desperately need to be better than everyone else.
- I feel a desperate inner panic and start holding my breath and can't think, though my mind is rushing a mile a minute.
- On the outside, I appear calm and collected, but inside I feel like I am in deep water, sinking.
- My normal response has been anger, frustration, cursing, bitterness, and the need to control or fix the situation. My surviving self wants to control everything because I don't ever feel safe.
- I jump to conclusions because I need to be right. But I am finding that I am wrong a lot. My surviving self feels less-than if I don't have all the answers.
- I define myself based on my financial wherewithal and zip code. My surviving self dresses up the outside because inside my life is a mess.
- When I feel like I'm in an environment where I'm not enough or I can't express myself, I become quiet and feel fear, doubt, and nervousness. I feel incapable. My surviving self never feels like I am enough.
- My heart races in a way that makes me feel at risk. My

surviving self is running fast. I feel like I'll fall apart if I slow down.

- I talk really fast because I am afraid of being interrupted or cut off. I am surviving by compensating for not being listened to or valued as a child.

What are your surviving self telltale signs, and what are you surviving?

Seeing the habits of our surviving self is the critical step we must take to reclaim ourselves as whole. Once we see our limiting thinking or behaviors and how they taunt and control us, we can't unsee them—and that's a good thing. They are forever exposed to the light of awareness that paves a path to healing. To get there, we must challenge our habits and reach for freedom.

ACCEPT THE SURVIVING SELF

Initially, I thought if I could just get rid of surviving self characteristics like focusing on what's wrong or being afraid of being hurt, I could live life more boldly. But the more I replayed the Dream of Self in my mind, the more I realized that recognizing the whole Self—the surviving self, the thriving Self, and the infinite SELF, working in balanced harmony—requires accepting all three.

The infinite SELF had patiently stood before the arguing, surviving self and listened without judgment, then stepped forward and wrapped the surviving self in her arms as it struggled with life. How many times did I attack my surviving self, thinking I needed to fix that part of me, or be smarter, or just be different? I was so busy blaming and vilifying the surviving self, I was unable to see the value it brings to my life. I wanted to wrap my arms around myself and assure the scared or flailing part of me that I was safe and connected to a great inner force that loved me unconditionally.

I thought about my parents and how I never had to barter for their love. They never once tried to reshape me into their vision of me, nor compared us siblings. They were patient as I tried to figure life out.

I felt respected. They disciplined me as needed, but they never withheld their love for any reason—not when I stole candy from the local store, lied about my whereabouts, dropped out of college, or had sex for the first time. Their love was unconditional. My gut told me that this was the kind of love I owed my Self, and that understanding the surviving self and having compassion for this part of me required that I treat it with the unconditional love my parents had shown me. Intuition said this was the road to inner stability and freedom.

I wanted to love my surviving self the way the compelling woman in my dream loved the flailing-arms woman and show compassion for the struggling parts of myself. These were new thoughts. I needed to discover what that looked like.

I found myself contemplating this conundrum: If the infinite SELF is as innate as the surviving self, then the surviving self serves an important role that needs to be understood and honored. I began to say to myself: *I want to see and understand my surviving self.*

Say:
I want to see and understand my surviving self.

The question of how to transform my relationship with my surviving self turned into a constant curiosity that changed how I worked with myself. My desire to skillfully work with the surviving self eventually birthed the **14 Practices for Inner Health and Well-being** offered in this book.

Ask:
How can I see and understand my surviving self?

WHAT ABOUT HAPPINESS?

In my work, a participant inevitably asks about the surviving self's ability to be happy.

I share this analogy: Imagine you are running for your life. Are you thinking about happiness? No. The fear of the surviving self denies access to the higher range of Self. Science tells us that when we are in survival mode—"Fight, flight, or freeze"—the body automatically shuts down unnecessary functions, such as digestion; shifts from relaxed to focused and mobilized; and redirects all available energy to the body's limbs to support running, fighting, or otherwise eluding danger.

Neither happiness nor concern for others is a consideration or concern of the surviving self. Its primary goal is survival, at whatever cost. The surviving self seeks safety. This means we will choose what is known and familiar over the unknown because we know how to survive the known and familiar, even if it is abusive or makes us unhappy. Often, we choose our partners and mates on the basis of our surviving self's fears and needs, because we don't yet have access to the empowering aspects of the thriving Self or infinite SELF.

Ask:
What is one thing I am surviving because it is my habit or comfort zone?

When we understand the nature of the surviving self, we can understand our choices. And what we see, we can change.

THE SURVIVING SELF RESISTS CHANGE

The aim of the surviving self in my Dream of Self, flailing her arms and stomping her feet on the beach, was to distract me from connecting with the compelling infinite SELF. I realized the surviving self can somehow sense when change is coming and fight against it. This is why our outdated beliefs and behaviors are so resistant to change.

I thought about the numerous times when I committed to a physical fitness routine or desired to change my attitude and met with inner resistance that sought to pull me back to my previous weight or attitude "set point." I didn't have words or any scientific insight to confirm this, but meeting with resistance was a consistent experience; resistance and the surviving self were the same. I paid attention to resistance wherever it showed up and reminded myself to look through it to the goal or life that was calling to me. I was learning to ignore resistance and trust the determination and ability of the whole Self to reconstruct itself and thrive.

Once I realized that this set-point dynamic was real, it could no longer unconsciously infiltrate my life. When resistance kicked in, I would employ the tool of *I See You* and see the resistance for what it was—an old, comfortable part of me fighting for its life. Old ideas, ways of behaving, reactions, ways we come to know ourselves, ways we want the world to see us, insecurities, and hopes fight to stay alive because *everything* wants to live.

 A Tool: I See You

I See You helps you see habits you want to break and habits you want to enforce and puts you in a more conscious and empowered relationship with your Self. When you uncover surviving self behavior that no longer serves you and you want to change your relationship to that behavior, say *I See You* to that behavior. This simple act shines a light on behavior that previously operated unseen.

Awareness is the beginning of the end for unconscious and unwanted behavior. *I See You* won't change unwanted behavior overnight; however, once the unconscious behavior is exposed to your awareness, its days are numbered. The more you see it, the less it can unconsciously live unchecked in your life.

When we begin to prioritize having a healthy relationship with our Self, the more we see ourselves doing things that don't serve or honor us, and the less willing we are to indulge in these old ways. Saying *I See You* to that behavior interrupts the unconscious, unsupportive behavior of the surviving self and gives you choices. When we see ourselves less triggered or judgmental, that's an occasion to say *I See You* to the thriving Self. The more we acknowledge our positive changes, the more conscious we become of the behavior that brings about change. That's the behavior we want to practice, practice, practice.

Some people are so distracted by their surviving self tendencies that they miss countless opportunities to see the good things in their lives and feel supported by the universe. Say *I See You* to the infinite SELF when an answer you need shows up, or when the person you need to talk to calls "out of the blue," or when the hurtful behavior of others doesn't affect you. These are opportunities to say *I See You* to your higher power.

EVERYTHING WANTS TO LIVE

I started wondering whether it was possible that a level of intelligence lives in everything. Going forward, when I wanted to grow or change, the intention I wrote down to help guide me would include being mindful of the future resistance that I was sure to meet.

Example: I set the intention to transform my judgmental thinking. Then, I'd ask an effective and empowering question (EEQ)—

how, what, who, or *where*—to help me see and move beyond any resistance that might try to stand in my way.

Ask:

How can I see any resistance that stands in my way and transform it with grace and ease?

Taking time to envision what I want, write it down, and anticipate the habitual surviving self resistance that would probably show up allowed me to consciously engage with the surviving self.

THE SCIENCE DEMANDS RESPECT

Scientific inquiry has determined that the brain constantly scans our environment for potential danger as part of its evolutionary programming. Our primitive ancestors had to be able to register threats quickly to avoid danger and increase their survival. Individuals who were more attuned to danger stayed alive longer and passed on their genes. You and I received those genes. As part of our DNA, we default to looking for what is wrong, feels unsafe, or threatens our existence. Without the tenacity of the surviving self and its ability to sense danger and evade it, you and I would not be here.

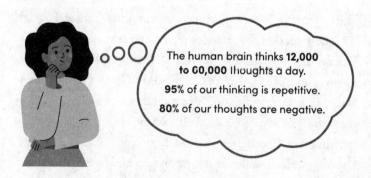

The human brain thinks **12,000 to 60,000** thoughts a day.

95% of our thinking is repetitive.

80% of our thoughts are negative.

We think thousands of thoughts daily. A 2020 study estimated we have six thousand thoughts a day, though some sources on the internet pose as many as sixty thousand. And most of those thoughts are negative and repetitive. This negativity bias shouldn't be surprising. For millions of years, humans have survived by focusing on and eluding problems and danger. The surviving self plays an important role in our evolution and deserves our respect and appreciation.

Today, due to the neocortex's development and the brain's executive management abilities, we can mitigate the negativity bias. We can consciously work with the brain's aspects that positively impact our lives.

Say:
My surviving self makes me human.
I can learn to understand my surviving self and work
deliberately with the thriving Self and infinite SELF.

The effective and empowering question "How do I transform my relationship with the surviving self?" makes room for the thriving Self to enter and empower our lives.

A Not-So-Random Story About Connection to the Unseen

Thirty years ago, at a spiritual consciousness course I took, the guest speaker for the closing session was named Juanita Dunn—a stately, sagelike woman with slow, deliberate movements and speech patterns. She said "Good evening" and launched into a fascinating story about an heirloom bracelet she wore and rarely took off. It had belonged to her great-grandmother. She shared that while sleeping during a trip to Las Vegas, the bracelet began to disturb her. In her sleep, she took the bracelet off and tucked it under her pillow, making a mental note to retrieve it in the morning.

It wasn't until she and her husband had driven halfway back to Los Angeles that she realized she was not wearing the bracelet. She then remembered the mental note she had made in her sleep and panicked. Back then, cell phones were not like pocket change; she couldn't just pull out a phone and alert the hotel. She had to wait until she got home. But when she spoke with the hotel, they said her heirloom bracelet was nowhere to be found.

She told the class that the idea that her bracelet was forever gone was unacceptable. Instead of sorrow and grief, she became filled with determination and single-mindedness. She made the decision that she was unwilling to be separated from that bracelet. She touched her right arm where the bracelet had rested for years and committed to seeing it on her arm and feeling its presence until it returned.

Months went by. One evening, she and her husband went to see a play. They parked the car and began to walk to the theater when she realized she didn't have the tickets with her. She quickly returned to the car where the tickets had fallen between the seats. As she blindly felt for the tickets underneath the seat, her hand landed on something oddly familiar. When she pulled back her hand, in it was her bracelet.

That was the end of Juanita Dunn's story. She did not say another word. We were all hanging on her every breath waiting for the conclusion, waiting for her to explain her mistake. But she just sat down. The teacher of the class came forward. He asked the class, by a show of hands, how many of us students thought the bracelet had always been in the car and that Juanita was mistaken about when or where she had lost it. Most hands in the room went up. Mine did not. The instructor of the class ended with these words: "The degree that you can believe this story happened just as it was told is the same degree to which your life will respond to you!"

His words touched a frequency that resonated throughout my entire body. I knew then, and I know now, that our connection to the unseen is unquestionable. From then until now, I constantly reach beyond my boundaries seeking to discover more about this wondrous universe that is our home. I expect to see what I have not been able to see up until the present moment. But I don't believe in miracles. I believe there is more to life than our current brain wiring can see or understand. I use effective and empowering questions to seek answers. I ask because asking makes room in my consciousness for an idea that is already possible, or I would not have been able to conceive such an idea. I also commit 1,000 percent to doing my best to figure things out. I don't see myself as Aladdin and the universe as the Genie. I see a partnership. My role is to make room inside of myself for answers that will come. I do this by wanting, and then servicing my want with new actions as best I can. This effort makes me more open, welcoming, and magnetic and fosters a relationship with possibility and the unseen and mystical process of creation.

The Thriving Self

The thriving Self is aware and proactive. It is the inner visionary and conduit to our higher power and all that is possible within us. In my Dream of Self, this Self constantly moves forward on the beach of life, seeing life as a teacher and using life events to grow and expand. The characteristics of the thriving Self make us resilient, capable of rising above circumstances, and empowered to change our lives. When the heart is filled with thriving Self qualities like hope, possibility, empathy, and gratitude, it becomes an open lane for the infinite SELF to freely move through. It helps us see ourselves as innately worthy and know we are capable and connected to something more powerful than our anxious thoughts and difficult circumstances.

The role of the thriving Self physiologically aligns with the operation of the frontal lobe of our brain, allowing us to be Self-aware, to reason, and to objectively observe, evaluate, and regulate our thinking and behavior.

The mindset of the thriving Self is: *Something new is possible, and life requires me to expand.*

SEEING MY THRIVING SELF

I returned to my Dream of Self to discover the characteristics and lessons of the thriving Self and the power of being curious. In recounting my dream, I referred to the main character as the Dreamer. However, I once read that all dreams and the people in them are about the person and life of the person who is dreaming—I realized that *I* was the Dreamer.

The dream began with me, as the thriving Self, walking up a secluded beach. Seeing this excited me. In the dream, I was being aware and proactive, moving forward, and focused on what was in front of me instead of behind me. I was in a contemplative mood—spending quality time with my thoughts. Indeed, this contemplativeness had entered my daily life; I was learning to let go of the past, be in the present moment, and dare to uncover new possibilities. Spending reflective time with my Self and practicing new behavior was changing my life. I was starting to see my surviving self in my awake life as clearly as the flailing arms of the woman on the beach in the dream.

In the dream, I was aware of my surroundings and noticed the two women arguing. A year or two earlier, politeness or concerns for safety would have led me to turn around and head in the opposite direction, but in the dream, I didn't turn back. Seeing this taught me that default habits no longer had to rule my life. Our ability to change is the power that the thriving Self adds to our lives. I was listening to my Self and following my intuition.

At any point or age in our lives, we can acknowledge how life has been and decide to change. Instead of adjusting myself to make others comfortable, I moved forward toward what was calling me. Curiosity grabbed with the force of a magnet. It pulled me to the two women on the beach and to an experience that would provide answers I'd been looking for my entire life.

As my surviving self saw me approach, her gesticulations intensified, but I was not distracted by her drama, even as her voice became louder. Her behavior could not pierce the connection that had formed between me and the compelling woman before me. I knew paying more attention to this part of my Self and less to the surviving self was an answer to the question *How do I become more of my Self?* My eyes were locked on the compelling woman, and I knew she saw me.

I objectively observed the two women before me: When the compelling one looked at me and then stepped toward the argumentative woman and hugged her, she sent a message of Self-acceptance and Self-love that changed my life. The safety and trust in their embrace allowed me, as the surviving self, to stop fighting and realize I was more than my habitual anger, worry, doubt, and fear. In the arms of the infinite SELF, I was secure and protected.

A CONDUIT

When the embracing women turned and looked at me, I was shocked and relieved to see they both were me. The one with her back to the ocean was the surviving self, driven by habit, and the one facing the ocean was the infinite SELF, a compelling presence and harbor of peace. I was in the middle with the ability to choose the safety of the known past, full of worry, doubt, and fear, or to trust in the elevated nature of a higher force. I saw that the thriving Self was a conduit between worry, doubt, and fear and peace and safety.

The thriving Self is the part of us that knows and chooses higher ground. No matter how ingrained a behavior or belief may be, the thriving Self provides the Self-agency necessary to act in advance of our historical reactions. This means that within us is the ability to make new choices regardless of our circumstances or how ingrained our responses. Despite my habit of worry, doubt, fear, and flailing my arms, I could learn to shift my thinking and thereby access more of my thriving Self.

 A Tool: Shifting Your Focus

Shifting your focus is a powerful mental tool that helps you stop defaulting to worry, doubt, fear, insecurity, and all their cousins. Shifting teaches you to tell your mind, *No! I will think about what's possible instead of hanging out in habitual worry, doubt, and fear.*

Like any practice, learning to shift your thinking takes time and repetition. But every time you deliberately manage the mind, you undermine its ingrained tendencies with new behavior that, with repetition, becomes a new habit. Considering what is possible rather than defaulting to the old habit leaves space inside our thinking for new ideas and choices. Sometimes it takes great effort to grab hold of the mind and shift. In the beginning, you might have to shift your thinking a thousand times a minute because the mind defaults to what it knows.

To experience the effort you must make, try this exercise: Stretch your arms out to the left of you, with your fists balled, like you're gripping something tightly. Then, with a little grunt that represents effort, and maintaining outstretched arms and balled-up fists, *shift* your arms to the right, like you are moving a rusted lever from left to right. It might take this kind of effort to shift your thoughts from negative tendencies at first. But the effort disrupts the habit, and disrupting the habit makes change possible.

THE POWER TO DISRUPT

The thriving Self is aware of the surviving self and has the power to interrupt our surviving self habits and move our thinking to higher ground. The surviving self exists within a limited perspective, unaware of its thriving Self and infinite SELF range. It doesn't realize it can resist the tendency to repetitively engage with negative thoughts.

I remember standing on that stage in the fifth grade, so terrified that I could not see or hear. The overwhelm felt endless, though the entire traumatic experience lasted maybe five minutes. But during those five minutes, there was nothing but fear and darkness, no hope or sense of possibility or future. When we are controlled by the surviving self, especially during a fight, flight, or freeze episode, we don't know another reality exists, and we can't access our imagination unless our thriving Self steps in, *shifts* our thinking to a more elevated state, and broadens our sense of Self. This is why building a strong thriving Self is crucial. A thriving mindset uses our connection to the infinite SELF to pull the surviving self to higher ground.

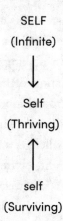

SELF
(Infinite)

Self
(Thriving)

self
(Surviving)

THE THRIVING SELF ALIGNS WITH SCIENCE

In his book *Cosmos,* American astronomer Carl Sagan wrote of the way he perceived the brain:

> Deep inside the skull of every one of us there is something like a brain of a crocodile. Surrounding the R-complex [the reptilian or lizard brain] is the limbic system or mammalian brain, which evolved tens of millions of years ago in ancestors who were mammal but not yet primates. It is a major source of our moods and emotions, of our concern and care for the young. And finally, on the outside, living in uneasy truce with the more primitive brains beneath, is the cerebral cortex; civilization is a product of the cerebral cortex.

I see the Three Selves in Sagan's way of seeing the brain: The reptilian brain is the surviving self, the frontal lobe is the thriving Self, and Sagan's exploration of the universe nods to the infinite SELF.

Human evolution took a leap forward with the development of the neocortex, which gives us the ability to imagine. According to an article by Amy F. T. Arnsten, this allows us "to plan and organize for the future," observe ourselves consciously and objectively, execute higher-order decision-making, and "orchestrate the brain's activity for intelligent regulation of behavior, thought, and emotion." The functions of the frontal lobe of the neocortex make the notion of a thriving Self real. The thriving Self can choose thoughts, imagine the future, plan, challenge, and change our lives beyond the danger-focused fight, flight, or freeze nature of the surviving self. The frontal lobe makes us a powerful species. The thriving Self makes us powerful in our individual lives, allowing us to see the surviving self and rise above its nature.

WHY WE NEED THE THRIVING SELF

When I read the above quotation from Sagan and came across the idea of the triune brain, I got excited. It instigated this insight regarding the Three Selves:

- The infinite SELF is the life from which all emerges. It is all, and therefore, **all is connected.**
- The thriving Self is aware of the surviving self and seeks connection to the infinite SELF.
- The surviving self sees only its needs, doubts, and fears.

The surviving self can't see beyond its nature. This is why people stuck in behaviors such as "othering" and assuming the worst treat other people so poorly. "Againstness" and distrust are second nature to the surviving self. When we are in survival mode, we project our surviving self mindset onto others. This is what makes the thriving Self so crucial. The thriving mindset brings Self-awareness to the surviving self and expands it beyond its limiting behavior.

THRIVING SELF QUALITIES

Abundance	Belief in Good	Expectation	Faith
Acceptance	Awareness	Compassion	Grace
Appreciation	Enthusiasm	Curiosity	Excitement	Forgiveness

Strengthen Your Thriving Self

The thriving Self gives us the ability to hope, dream, and make new choices. With the thriving Self we see ourselves as connected to something more powerful than our anxious thoughts. Here are the ways the thriving Self shows up in our lives.

Gratitude	Freedom	Openness	Trust	Thanksgiving
Hope	Self-Love	Optimism	Unity
Inspiration	Joy	Possibility	Vulnerability

The thriving Self is named for its thriving qualities and traits that elevate our thinking and feelings. There's a powerful openness and sense of possibility in thriving characteristics. I began to pay attention to what made me feel empowered and capable and thereby expanded my list of thriving characteristics. Other thriving Self qualities I began to pay attention to were the choices to be curious, desire and ask for support, leave room in my thinking for the infinite intelligence, and courageously move forward, change directions, or not. The more I contemplated my power to choose, the more my personal power emerged.

The thriving Self trusts that it is connected to the infinite SELF and therefore feels safe in the world, not because of who it knows or its financial means; rather, it trusts its connection to the infinite life source. This knowing distinguishes it from the surviving self. The thriving Self engages with challenges and discomfort with acceptance, understanding that discomfort comes with creation and difficulty is the tunnel we travel to opportunity.

When faced with difficulty, I visit the list of thriving Self qualities and choose one, or a few, to guide my thinking and behavior to maintain an elevated, clear-thinking approach. If I see myself thinking about worst-case scenarios, I use the tool of shifting my focus and shift to thinking about the good that is possible. The list of thriving Self characteristics encourages optimism and reminds me to elevate my thoughts, act faithfully, and choose to believe that good is available in every situation. This behavior aligns with research by neuroscientist Tali Sharot, who writes about what she calls the "optimism bias." She says, "Hope focuses on wanting something and optimism elevates hope to the belief that what you want is likely to happen. If you think something can lead to good, you are more likely to take action that supports your belief in the likelihood." When we shift our thinking, our expectations impact our actions, and our actions impact our outcomes.

In the days, weeks, and years following my Dream of Self, I've developed an intricate understanding of the thriving Self. Today I know this part of each of us is more powerful than the surviving self. The audacity of hope is, indeed, powerful. This is the part of us that wisely dares to hope against all odds and uses every situation and circumstance to move closer to the infinite SELF.

Say:
Engaging with hope and a sense of possibility will change my life for the better.

The Infinite SELF

The infinite SELF is the eternal, unwavering existence permeating all life, including every human being; it is present in the background of every moment and circumstance and is the space between everything that connects it all. The space in the infinite SELF is never empty. It is full of life and intelligence. It is the starting point of life. From here, everything emerges into life and returns from it. The infinite SELF is the universal power that goes by whatever name you use for your higher power. It doesn't just live in the world; it lives inside of every human and all life.

The mindset of the infinite SELF is: *I am the ever-expanding force behind life; I use life to reveal more of my endless potential.*

A CARING PRESENCE

My favorite moment in the Dream of Self is when the infinite SELF steps forward and, with a calming hug, penetrates the surviving self's arguing nature, and the surviving self releases her fight and fear and relaxes into the arms of her infinite SELF.

I knew that such care was possible.

I have experienced many mystical instances of feeling protected and guided by a force greater than myself. Once in my twenties, when I lived in that five-hundred-square-foot studio apartment, I was sleeping and heard someone sweetly yet commandingly call my name. I heard my name called three times before I entirely woke up. I opened my eyes and said "What?" at the same time. No one was in the apartment with me, yet just before I opened my eyes, I felt a hand touch my shoulder and shake me. Through the doorway to the kitchenette, I saw an orange glow and heard a popping sound. I jumped up and ran to the kitchen. A pan of cooking oil on the stove was in flames because I had forgotten to turn off the burner. What woke me up? How did I hear a voice when no one was in the room?

We all have received support and care from the infinite universe whether we were sensitive to this phenomenon or not. We are a part of an intelligent, unwavering presence and power that connects and expresses through all. The DNA of this cosmic force animates life. This presence as the foundational structure of our lives makes us more than any label or circumstance because the whole of anything is always greater than its parts. No matter how devastating an event is or how much we struggle emotionally, the unseen presence of the infinite SELF makes us more than an idea, feeling, or event. I knew that strengthening my connection to this SELF would allow me to remember that my essence is more than any challenge I face when life bumps into me.

THE FORCE IS ALWAYS PRESENT

Believing "in" something is different from being one with it. Believing in a higher power or even believing in ourselves means two things are present—us and the thing we believe in. If I can believe in something, I can also choose to not believe in it. I was no longer willing to think in terms of separation—me and a higher power. This view is flawed. Life is a package deal; with life comes the force that makes life possible.

I wanted to live my life with an inner knowing that the inner Self, which is the essence of me, is greater than external circumstances. I wanted to know that in me dwells a life—bigger, stronger, and more powerful—that makes my life possible and that fosters my growth. I wanted to trust that feelings like inadequacy, shame, and insecurity stretch and break as the great life within emerges. I was ready to learn the skills and practices that foster a conscious connection with this limitless force. I wanted to be the compelling force in the Dream of Self that could stand in front of all parts of my Self and life, centered and whole.

If we are extensions of the limitless force behind all, there is more to us than the lies, limiting ideas, and experiences that shape or harass us. We must redefine ourselves not as the parts but as the whole, move the parts from center stage, and see the whole that holds the parts.

As I began to challenge my default to fear regarding my fifth-grade trauma, two simple mindset strategies helped create the internal space I needed for change to occur. First, during instances of internal doubt and resistance, I reminded myself often that in an infinite universe, there must be a way to achieve the things I want and transform the parts of me that cause me pain. This statement made sense to my brain and made room inside me for a new relationship with my Self. I told myself, *Yes, in an infinite universe, much more than I can imagine is possible.* This internal agreement left me believing change was possible. I dared to seek freedom even when I couldn't see it or I was triggered.

Say:
In an infinite universe, there must be a way to thrive beyond my challenges.

The second simple strategy is an inner fitness prompt I call **CREWW**—an acronym that further claims that the nature of the universe is our nature. CREWW helps us remember that we are innately Creative, Resilient, Empowered to choose, Whole, and Worthy.

Creative: You are the creative solution that can respond to any problem in a way that honors and affirms the Self. How you respond in any situation creates something. What are you creating?

Resilient: Your body, mind, and spirit are innately resilient. Maintaining inner alignment by acknowledging and honoring your inner Self activates resilience.

Empowered to choose: You always have the power to make a Self-empowering choice.

Whole: Your wholeness is measured not by body parts but by your ability to grow and make Self-empowering and Self-honoring choices that move you forward and keep you aligned with your inner Self and personal power.

Worthy: Your unique fingerprint confirms that you are intentionally designed. You are worthy because you exist.

In street parlance, *your CREWW always has your back.*

Think of CREWW as an internal posse. It stands up for the parts of ourselves that need our strength to heal, grow, and thrive. If there is an internal fight or an external confrontation with a person or group, our CREWW steps forward with force and presence to remind us that the infinite SELF dwells within and our greatest choice in any confrontation is to use the moment to grow and make Self-honoring choices. *When we let the surviving self dictate our actions, we cut ourselves off from our inner power and hand it over to external people and forces.* Regardless of the risk or fear we might feel, cultivating our whole Self demands that we honor our Self. Doing so gives us the opportunity to forge trust in our connection to something greater.

* * *

I was in a business setting once where I experienced sign after sign that I was being set up to be humiliated. I had studied narcissism, psychopathy, and Machiavellian personality types and had seen this kind of behavior before. I knew to be mindful of the gaslighting that is often associated with such personalities, and how these people are not done until they feel they have hurt you deeply. Such behavior can undermine one's sense of Self if one encounters it naively or unaware. But I knew to expect that some form of humiliation was methodically being orchestrated.

When the moment of intended humiliation occurred, I was meant to be minimized, to be made to feel nonexistent. The moment was masterfully cloaked to appear to be an innocent oversight instead of a deliberate message and insult.

I knew that making a Self-honoring choice at that moment was the most important choice of my life. I trusted that my CREWW would help me resiliently recover and that believing in a force greater than human beings would help me maintain the ultimate definition of being whole and worthy. So, rather than pretend nothing was happening and accept the gaslighting I was experiencing so that my ego could save face in front of a crowd of people, I spoke up. I made a Self-empowering choice without concern for the consequences.

When I tell this story, people ask me where my courage to speak up came from. I say, "My internal posse." I knew my CREWW had my back. Knowing that my life is supported by and aligned with a power greater than myself and that the way to honor that power is to honor my Self made my choice simple and automatic. In forging a CREWW mindset, we learn to honor the highest spiritual essence within us as our ultimate commitment, source, and resource. This mindset says that being aligned with the inner Self is more powerful than external ideas of power.

Take a moment:
Recall a time in your life, or someone else's, when you, or that other person, made an empowering Self-aligned choice despite external pressures.

I recommend adopting and memorizing the following statement to help you recondition your sense of Self to align more with the infinite SELF.

Say:
I am innately *creative* enough to design and redesign

my life, *resilient* enough to weather any storm,

empowered to choose and rechoose my choices,

mystically *worthy* and undeniably *whole* in the eyes

of the universal force that lives within me.

When you face difficulty, or as a general practice, you can use this truth statement to remind yourself of your core nature.

Pay attention to how the statement feels in your body. Stating this truth will give you flashes of peace and hope. With practice, those flashes will become a lifestyle. Connecting with a higher sense of Self makes room in an anxious mind for elevated thoughts and a sense of possibility. Engage with this statement often. It will help create space for more of its wisdom and truth to emerge.

Inner knowing is the journey I am on today and, I hope, for the rest of my life. In the Dream of Self, knowing was modeled by the compelling woman. Seeing her gave me something to aim for. A concrete idea formed. I wanted to make room in my life for knowing, trusting, and seeing my Self as being one with the universal force, and my life as always on purpose, and trust that something beautiful and necessary is being created however life bumps into me. The infinite SELF promises the ability to experience life's circumstances, yet not be defined by them. I wanted to effectively address the people and things that bumped into me without ever allowing them to define me or lie to me about who I am or what's possible for my life.

CREATING SPACE

I reasoned that if the infinite SELF represents the highest range of consciousness and it dwells within me, rather than as a bearded man in the sky, then learning to think and see differently was required. To achieve this, I had to reach for a higher level of consciousness. To think from a higher consciousness requires first connecting with the space inside of us through which a higher consciousness can emerge.

I began to deliberately challenge and elevate my thoughts. I turned to an adage I learned years earlier and to this day hold in my heart like a prayer: *When you believe more in what you don't see than in what you do see, then what you don't see, you will see, and what you do see, you won't see.* I experimented with finding or creating practices I could engage in that would help me stay open and available to a deeper inner journey and unshakable connection to my inner Self.

One of my daily go-to practices is to breathe deeply and, on the exhale, imagine my inner Self being as spacious as a night filled with stars. Going within in this way reminds me there is more to us than our physical bodies. There are times when the inner landscape feels as vast as the sky.

Another practice I've learned is adapted from the Trust Technique, a technique for changing the emotional state of animals that I find powerful as a practice for human Self-regulation: You become very still inside and bring a soft focus to an object while also being focused on a sound, such as your breathing. There is a difference between focusing in these ways and engaging in these ways. Engagement is active and leads to a mind crowded with thinking. But focus eliminates thinking. Stillness, coupled with focus, creates inner space. When thinking lessens or quiets, we become more spacious inside. There is more room for truth. The intelligence of the universe has space to emerge. This is why meditation and mindfulness are powerful tools.

My intuition told me that being in a more honest and connected relationship with my Self was a straight line to a stronger relationship with the infinite SELF. When difficulty, confusion, or need of any kind surfaced, I would have full-blown audible conversations with this invisible presence that permeates all— sharing my feelings and asking for support and guidance. I would ask effective and empowering questions such as *What should I do? What is the best way to think of this? What would you have me do?* By asking questions, we acknowledge that a higher consciousness and other possibilities exist and open ourselves to expanding beyond where we are. I didn't have to know what the higher thought was. I just needed to acknowledge there was one and reach beyond where I was.

This optimism creates a doorway for answers to come into our lives. Like a mantra, I began to ask, "What higher thought can I think in this situation?" no matter the nature of the situation. This is how I began to realize my ability to default to the mindset that I am more than any circumstance I face.

GROWTH, EXPANSION, AND INNER SPACE

One day, while I was meditating, I saw an endless vine of green leaves. At first, I didn't think much of the vision. But I remembered the vine while staring out my window thinking about how the universe began as a tiny dot that keeps expanding. From that dot everything we see has emerged. One scientific theory says that enfolded within that original tiny dot was and is the unfolding universe. This thought floated into my mind: *If we are a microcosm of the universe, then its nature is our nature.* I began to contemplate what I knew about the universe. It wasn't a lot. But three features stood out as undeniable: The universe constantly expands and reveals more of itself; all life grows or replicates in number, like cells; and growth and expansion require space.

As I contemplated growth, expansion, and space, people I knew who were unhappy came to mind. I saw in them an avoidance or unwillingness to grow, or a fear of stepping into unknown territory, or a refusal to expand their thinking and explore new ideas. They were full of worry, doubt, fear, the need to control, and sad memories or stories. There was no space for something more. It occurred to me that *maybe our innate purpose is to grow and expand like the universe does.* This thought stuck.

The infinite SELF is intentional. And, like every fingerprint is unique and every cell in the body has a role to play, each of us has come into manifestation for a certain purpose **that fulfills the intention of the infinite SELF.** Indian sage Ramana Maharshi said, "The purpose of [your] birth will be fulfilled whether you will it or not."

If life is intentional in its journey and we have a role in the journey whether we are aware of the role or not, then we are innately purposeful whether we are aware of this or not. Each person matters in the body of the unfolding infinite SELF. Our purpose is to grow, expand, and create more space for the infinite SELF to live through us. We align with the infinite when we include the infinite SELF in our sense of Self. Our career, family, and station in life are only the court or field on which we play life. But to truly fulfill our lives and honor the Self, we must use our circumstances to expand the inner Self. Just as the universe expands and reveals more life, more of who you are waits beyond your limiting thoughts, feelings, and beliefs. Expanding one's consciousness gives the infinite SELF a seat at the center of our soul.

Say:

I am the ever-expanding harmonious nature of life.

Life uses me to grow, expand, and reveal more of its endless potential to the degree that I allow.

In my Dream of Self, I saw growth, expansion, and space throughout the dream. The compelling woman facing the argumentative woman was also facing the endless ocean and boundless sky. She was infinity facing infinity. The waves rushed to life and then disappeared. She never said a word. She didn't have to. Her presence was profound and loud.

The compelling woman compassionately stood before the argumentative woman, fully present, listening without a drop of judgment; she modeled for me how to transform my life by being present, seeing myself in others, and listening. She then did two things that changed me forever: She looked at me as though she knew everything about me, and then she turned her gaze onto the quarreling woman, stepped in, and hugged her. I would learn to do this with myself more.

This is how I would grow and expand into my Self. When both women turned and looked at me, I felt that the universe had orchestrated this moment and used these women to model a choice I could make throughout the rest of my life: trust myself enough to know my Self, step in, and hold myself close to the truth. The presence of the infinite SELF and her love made space for the surviving self to relax and open. From here the conscious union with SELF occurred.

Ask:
How must I grow and expand to thrive?

I woke from the dream driven to embrace the infinite SELF within. All sacred writings and wisdom have made their way into the world through people who stretched to hear the SELF. I would live out my purpose by strengthening my connection to the SELF, trusting its presence to navigate life and maintain harmony with my

Self. With this revelation, I no longer had to look for my purpose. I was standing in it: I must fill myself with better thoughts, challenge my beliefs, monitor my behavior, and cultivate space within to grow and expand.

Ask:

What must I do and who must I become to access more of my Self?

THE THREE SELVES AT A GLANCE

Surviving self	Thriving Self	Infinite SELF
Doubt	Optimism	The source and essence of all creation
Judgment	Acceptance	
Lack	Abundance	Love
Blame	Hope/Possibility	
Isolation	Trust	Inner spaciousness
Negativity	Gratitude	
Anger	Forgiveness	Cannot be hurt, harmed, or endangered
Hatred	Self-love	
Victimization	Freedom	Always expanding to reveal endless inner potential
Self-contraction	Self-expansion	

Know Thy Whole Self

T HE THREE SELVES SUPPORT THE JOURNEY OF KNOWING thy whole Self. Being able to see which self is driving your thoughts affects how you create and navigate your life. Since the time of the ancient Greeks, philosophers have encouraged us to "know thyself," to seek to see ourselves clearly and more deeply. The Dream of Self, and the 7 Laws of Self, invite you to view your Self with greater understanding and reverence.

In our effort to know our whole Self, we must learn to be more trusting and deliberate about how we see and treat ourselves, understand the fear and resistance that the surviving self defaults to, and not take it personally. We must practice shifting our thinking from thoughts of survival to thriving and thereby transform fear with understanding and profound Self-acceptance. And when life bumps into us, we must use it to make ourselves better. This is how we embrace our whole Self, grow and expand, and leave space for the infinite to emerge.

For years, I longed for practical and reliable steps to connect more deeply with my inner Self. One day, while flipping through my journals from the past twenty-five to thirty years, I noticed the phrase "remember this" written in the margins repeatedly. It urged me to memorize the empowering actions I had taken and the transformational insights I had gained. As an exercise, I compiled these notes into a document. Upon reading through them, I realized that many conveyed similar themes, revealing a set of go-to practices—intentional ways of thinking and behaving that could keep me grounded and aligned.

This experience inspired me to create the 14 Practices for Inner Health and Wellbeing, which I am excited to share now. These practices are not just ideas but practical tools you can revisit, engage with, and depend on as you cultivate a relationship with your inner Self.

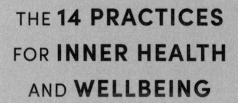

THE **14 PRACTICES** FOR **INNER HEALTH** AND **WELLBEING**

*The first step to feeling better
is knowing what to do.*

You Are Not Alone

———

*I practice turning my life over to a power greater
than me that loves me and responds to my heart.*

THIS PRACTICE WILL HELP YOU TO BE A PARTNER WITH the governing force behind life. It doesn't matter whether you come to this practice believing in a power greater than yourself or not. We all believe in something, and our beliefs drive our lives. Our thoughts, feelings, actions, and reactions are creative in nature, as is the universe. This places us in an active partnership with life. Practice 1—*I practice turning my life over to a power greater than me that loves me and responds to my heart*—will help you consciously engage with the universe and actively trust that "something" sees and responds to you.

There's Something Bigger

The intelligent force behind life holds the planets in place and supports the automatic functions of the human body. It also powers our intuition and makes profound love, joy, and forgiveness possible. By becoming curious about this force, I have experienced a softening of my heart and been filled with forgiveness that I did not know I wanted or think was possible. Where do such "bigger than us" moments and experiences come from? The infinite SELF is the door through which these experiences enter our lives.

Acknowledging that there is more within us than our pettiness and limitations opens our consciousness to seeing the greater range of the Self that dwells within.

The force behind life can be called many things: higher power, universal intelligence, spirit, infinite SELF, God, Yahweh, Jesus, Buddha, Allah, Krishna, Brahman, to name a few. Over the years, I've heard God lovingly referred to as Father, Mother, Brother, Bro, and Tree. In developing *your* relationship with your higher power, the name you use is up to you. The name that someone else chooses to use is their business. The name is not the point. Focusing on a name takes our eyes off the prize: seeing this higher force as an active part of our lives and building a one-on-one relationship that takes the force out of the heavens and places it inside our everyday lives.

A Not-So-Random Story About a Greater Power

Decades ago, I was working as a secretary for a small celebrity publicist. One particular late afternoon, she came to my desk and said, "Tomorrow, I won't be in until the afternoon." Then she left the office for the evening. Because our relationship had become strained, my intuition told me that her statement was a setup. I felt in my gut that she was going to call the office at 9:00 a.m., and if I was not there, she would fire me. I needed to give myself plenty of time. I got up extra early the following morning. I could not risk being even five minutes late, as I was often ten minutes late. My car was at the repair shop, so I would have to take two buses and walk about half a mile. Half a mile in I realized that my keys to the office were at home on my car key ring. My heart began to race. It was close to 9:00 a.m., and I had no way of getting into the office. Everything that happened next felt like I was watching a movie versus living the experience. I started walking really fast toward the office, then running. My mind was conjuring images of ladders, open second-floor windows, ajar doors, or maybe the building owner, who didn't live on the property, would magically appear. Internally, I was exploding. It felt like a cross between an electrical storm and fireworks going off inside me. I was going to be in that office when the phone rang.

Fifty yards from the office stairwell I saw something shiny. As I got closer, my gut knew it was a key. When I reached the stairwell, there was a key in the middle of the first step. Again, intuition told me the key was going to open the door. The phone started to ring. It was 9:00 a.m. on the nose. I ran up the stairs and shoved the key in the lock perfectly on the first try. I turned the key, and the door opened. I answered the phone; it was my boss. I heard the surprise in her voice. We talked briefly. Before we hung up, I asked her if she had her keys. She said yes. I hung up the phone in quiet awe. What had just happened? My gut knew: *A power greater than me had responded to my heart.*

Say:

Up until now, I've seen my Self and life one way, but from this point forward my vision can expand.

You Matter

If a force runs through *all*, "all" includes you. It is impossible to separate the force behind life from the life it creates. That would be like trying to make a distinction between sand and grains of sand. They are one and the same. If the force that sustains the universe lives within you, then you are made from the force, and therefore you carry its essence and creative nature. You, my friend, are holy ground. Take that in. You have access to as much or as little of the force as you can tune in to and can turn to it at any point; it is always there, fully present.

I trust that you or someone you know has experienced a miraculous story, received a much-needed answer, or had a person or event enter your life at the "perfect" time. What orchestrates such tailor-made moments? How is it that someone calls you and says exactly what you need to hear when you need it most? What is this phenomenon that brings into your life the things you need and long for? Life is responding this way all over the planet. These moments are often labeled "coincidences" until we learn to see them as proof that we are not alone in this world. We matter. Something responds.

Such mystical occurrences visit us common folk as often as they visit mystics. The difference between us and the mystics is that mystics look for and expect to see the force in everything. They know the force is present in every molecule of life and are eager to see this higher power in, through, and around all things.

We learn to trust that we matter by paying attention and acknowledging the care-filled moments that enter our lives. When we can see the universe winking at us through a stream of green lights when we're driving in a hurry or that one available parking space when we're running late, we learn to ask for support regarding our more important needs.

When we feel we matter and are in partnership with a higher power, we can dare to challenge unchallenged areas of our lives and expect new possibilities. This is the thriving Self in action.

Practice 1—*I practice turning my life over to a power greater than me that loves me and responds to my heart*—is where you start. This affirms the reality of the partnership between you and the greater force. This is a bold starting point because it inserts you into the cosmic tapestry. It says that the universe responds to your thoughts and feelings.

This means you matter. You make a difference, and how you think and feel impacts life. This makes you a creator working within the creative nature of life. Life is not just bumping into you, spinning you in one direction and then the next. You are also bumping into life and reshaping it. Your thoughts, feelings, beliefs, actions, and reactions mold and reshape your experiences.

You can be intentional about what you hold in your mind and heart. When the creative nature of life meets your intentionality, you and the universe create together. This is what has been missing from your idea of yourself—the ability to see yourself as a partner in life with your higher power. Wherever you go, there, too, is your partner and the full power of the universe.

What's in Your Heart Matters

If the force responds to our hearts, then we must be mindful of what lives in our minds and hearts. When we choose to see ourselves as powerless, broken, or unlucky, we choose to worry, doubt, fear, and constantly feel at risk. This is an example of operating from the surviving self.

Reclaiming ourselves requires us to fill our minds and hearts with better visions and possibilities for our lives, and to lead with a sense of possibility and hope. This is work the thriving Self can achieve. The surviving self does what is safe and familiar. The thriving Self drives our ability to choose something better for our lives. We must envision the kind of person we want to be, the peace we wish to experience, and the sense of purposefulness we want to drive us. Remember the saying "We become what we think about all day long."

If surviving behavior fills the mind and heart with worry, doubt, and fear, and you are always at war in the world, you will generate and plant in the world more worry, doubt, fear, and war. However, when the thriving Self leads, the desire to grow and expand into more of yourself lives in your heart, and behaviors that support thriving will become your new actions. The power that responds to your heart does not police your thinking. It allows you to create your world according to your beliefs.

You must cultivate a mind and heart full of what you want and who you want to be rather than what you don't want, which disconnects you from your Self. This is your responsibility alone. No one can physically enter your mind and heart and change your thoughts and feelings. Changing your habit from one of judging yourself harshly and focusing on what is wrong to one of Self-acceptance and focusing on what's possible for you and your life takes personal **EFFORT** (Extracting Freedom From Our Restricted Thinking).

Turn *Effort* into a Verb

At first, this practice seems to be about faith—asking you to turn your life over to an unseen force. But look closer. You'll see this practice is about *efforting*, that is, *building* faith in your ability to live feeling connected to something greater.

It takes effort to not get distracted by day-to-day living, to think we can achieve more internal freedom, to pause when we're triggered, and to remember we can consciously use any moment to change our lives. It takes effort to try to be in a relationship with a force we cannot see or to believe we are seen and worthy of being responded to, and it takes effort to wrestle with the surviving self. All this effort can sound like too much if you define effort as only involving work.

But what happens if we see effort as the opportunity life provides for us to move toward freedom? This is the question that birthed my acronym EFFORT. Freedom lives jailed in us waiting to be set free. Up until now, our doubtful thinking and habitual ways of seeing ourselves and life has stood between us and the person we want to be and how we want to feel inside. But from this point forward, efforting to break free of our old thinking and patterns is how we free ourselves from limitations, learn, grow, and change. Effort is the path to freedom.

The dictionary defines *effort* as "a vigorously determined attempt." If we add the EFFORT acronym to the dictionary definition, we get this: *Effort—a vigorously determined attempt to extract freedom from our restricted thinking.* This is the effort change and growth require.

Effort is the action we take that makes room for faith. Earnestly "trying" is an action. Efforting to see past our blind spots and to think and react differently is a powerful action.

The surviving self pulls you in the direction of being afraid and closed and feeling like you must figure everything out on your own. The affirmation of Practice 1—*I practice turning my life over to a power greater than me that loves me and responds to my heart*—is full of actionable steps that counter surviving self tendencies: practice trying to see beyond your surviving self; practice trying to turn your life over to your higher power; practice trying to believe that a higher power loves you and responds to your heart; practice trying to believe you are worthy of this effort. When you expend the effort to turn these concepts into action, that effort develops inner fitness and opens you to receive.

Trying has but one rule: Put forth sincere effort. Your "try" might look different from another person's. You might throw your hands in the air and openheartedly say, *Show me God. Guide me. Lift me.* You might cry with frustration at what look like moments of failure and continue to try anyway. You might meditate, sing, or dance to extract freedom from your restricted habitual behaviors and ways. If you are reaching beyond a limitation, you are trying, and every effort is moving you closer to where you want to be. Consistent effort is the process. This is how trust in the partnership develops. Faith in something greater is the inevitable outcome.

Say:
Whatever EFFORT I make counts in the name of growing into more of my Self.

Unconditionally Present

You don't have to drop to your knees; believe despite your doubt; pray in hushed, reverent tones; or use a certain name for the force to respond. You can be full of doubt, angry, feeling forgotten, resistant, and even arrogant.

There is no bartering or quid pro quo in this practice. Whether you choose to turn your life over to a higher intelligence or not, that force is still in the back of your life unconditionally loving you and responding to your heart. It is up to you to flip the switch and see that your thoughts matter; what you carry in your heart is what the greater force responds to. From this vantage point, you can see how your thoughts, feelings, and beliefs matter—and that constantly exploring, weeding, and upgrading them also matters.

To feel better, do better, and be better, you must take ownership of your journey—acknowledge without judgment where you are and where you yearn to go. Spending this quality time with Self gives you greater clarity about everything: your tendency to doubt or hope, what you want or don't want, and what you don't know and yearn to know, or don't feel and yearn to feel. This clarity becomes the "stuff" that your higher power responds to.

YOU ARE NOT ALONE

A Revolutionary Act

Fall in love with putting forth the **EFFORT** (**E**xtracting **F**reedom **F**rom **O**ur **R**estricted **T**hinking) of honoring your Self and the greater force that loves you and responds to your heart.

Inner Fitness Opportunity

Faith and freedom

EEQ (Effective and Empowering Question)

Ask aloud:

How can I develop the faith to trust that my efforts will produce astounding results?

Ask for Assistance

I ask for my higher power's assistance in all I do.

Practice 1—*I practice turning my life over to a power greater than me that loves me and responds to my heart*—is partners with Practice 2—*I ask for my higher power's assistance in all I do*—and places you in an active relationship with your higher power.

Power Dwells Within

In every mature heart, unresolved hurt is waiting to heal, dreams are waiting to be fulfilled, and a force greater than you is present to support your effort. This is the state of being human. What good is a higher power if you don't seek its wisdom, guidance, and support and expect to receive it?

Don't give up your dreams simply because you don't know where to start or run from wanting more because it causes uncomfortable feelings. Leaving unaddressed dreams or hurt locked inside feels worse. Yes, not knowing where to start or how to move your life forward can feel lonely and overwhelming. But every dream and future version of you begins here.

Practice 2—*I ask for my higher power's assistance in all I do*—reminds you there is a force and a resource greater than you whose nature is to guide and support. Therefore, you are never alone in any moment or circumstance, nor do you have to figure life out all by yourself.

Your responsibility is to ask your higher power for assistance. The infinite SELF is the connection point between you and your higher power. Your **EFFORT** (Extracting Freedom From Our Restricted Thinking) is to develop this connection. *Asking for assistance in all that you do* brings your higher power out of the heavens and into your life. Exerting this effort makes room in your mind and heart for receiving.

Within the effort of asking, a part of you is saying, "I know more is possible; I know there is a way through this." When you stop to ask for assistance, your effort interrupts the negative tendencies of the mind and shifts you into the range of mind where your intention, feelings of hope and possibility, and vision of a better future have room to unfold.

Just Ask

We human beings complicate the simple age-old directive of "Ask and it shall be given." Instead of following this ancient wisdom, people come up with a list of reasons not to ask for assistance: They decide it is more spiritual not to ask; they don't want to "bother" or "insult" their God (as if either scenario is possible); or they make up their minds that asking is being needy or greedy. Proudly, they do everything by themselves because they've heard so often that the higher force "never gives us more than we can handle." They feel their higher power already knows what they want and need. Many are simply afraid to ask for fear of not getting what they ask for. There is so much confusion around this simple and direct advice: Ask.

This ancient teaching doesn't say ask for this or that only. It doesn't say you can ask only if you have been good and attend church regularly. Nor does it suggest you have to suffer first and then ask. It says ASK whenever you want to or need to. ASK for anything. No matter why you ASK, your ASK fosters connection.

Ask for qualities: I desire and ask for more freedom, trust, joy, abundance, or whatever in my life.

Ask for things: I desire and ask for a job that aligns with my purpose and allows me the joy of being well-paid for work I love.

Ask for transformation: I desire and ask for my pain and sadness to be transformed into peace and joy.

Ask for healing: I desire and ask that my body be strengthened and healed.

Ask for clarity: I desire and ask for the clarity that allows me to confidently make the decisions I need to make.

Ask for direction: I desire and ask that my next steps be made undeniably clear.

Ask for assistance.

Ask for freedom to be you!

ASK! ASK! ASK!

You can even ask to better understand the point I'm making here: *I ask to better understand what I've just read, heard, seen, or experienced.* There is no limit to what you can ask for—nor is there any limit to your higher power's ability to respond.

Asking your higher power for assistance in acknowledging your dreams and desires or achieving freedom from past hurt is a way to connect with your Self and strengthen your relationship with your higher power at the same time.

There Is More to Asking Than the Request

Asking is a powerful activity that builds the thriving Self.

When we ask for what we want, we consciously acknowledge the universal force behind life as the ultimate source of the support and fulfillment we desire and the ultimate supplier of our good. Asking is an act of surrender to a power greater than ourselves. It implies that we don't know how best to get what we want, but by asking, we are moved into the thriving Self where openness, curiosity, hope, and a sense of possibility dwell.

The effort of *asking for that higher power's assistance in all I do* moves you into a higher range of consciousness where the energy of a thriving mindset is activated.

Asking . . .

- acknowledges that a force greater than you is the orchestrating energy behind your life.
- trusts *something* is listening.
- affirms the responsive nature of the universe.
- assumes your worthiness.
- directs your focus and sets your intention.
- stimulates co-creation with a force greater than you.
- supports free will.
- allows you to acknowledge your human desire and spiritual expectations.
- allows you to be a student learning to trust in the nature of God/the universe.

- encourages conscious interaction with the "unseen" as being real.
- frees you from trying to figure out life on your own.
- practices courage and vulnerability.

Go Deeper

The *in all I do* portion of Practice 2 is particularly important. For a long time, I thought I had this practice mastered because I talk out loud to the universe all the time. Daily I say things like "Okay, God, what should I do here?" But when I engaged a deeper consideration of this practice, *in all I do* surprised me. I began to see many areas where I could ask for assistance but wasn't. Some areas had been a challenge for so long that unconsciously I had stopped expecting change or trying to change. Instead, I hid the challenge from the world and pretended I was okay.

I was leaving the force greater than me out of the areas where I needed the most help.

Asking for assistance *in all I do* encourages true partnership. It means bringing to the relationship your deepest vulnerability, insecurity, hope, or disappointment so that your relationship to your problems can change.

Say:

Up until now, an area where I have stopped expecting change is _____. But from this point forward I ASK that this area change for the better.

Ask for Everything

We're talking about not leaving any need or area of your life out: We can ask for assistance in that area where we have had the greatest amount of challenge; where an experience or memory still leaves us upset, feeling alone, or not good enough; or where there is a lack of forgiveness—ours or someone else's. We can ask for help with a challenge that has been with us so long that we've stopped believing there's anything we can do to change it.

Right there, where we've given up hope for things being different or better, we can ask for assistance. We can turn to our higher power and say out loud, "This thing that I have been carrying for such a long time, I ask you to please show me how to be free of it," or "I ask you to step into my life in this area and move me to a level of freedom and awareness and surrender where it no longer burdens me."

To *ask for that higher power's assistance in ALL I do* means there is no limit to what we can choose to ask for assistance with. Having a hard time falling asleep at night? "I ask the force greater than me to help me fall asleep" can be as effective as a sleeping pill. This sounds small, but I was excited when I discovered I could ask for help falling asleep, or even having an orgasm. Yep, you heard me right. Try this, and any other ask that comes to mind.

When you don't know which way to turn, what to do next, or how to free your Self from a stuck place, and you desire to move forward, to *ask* is *effort* that puts this practice to work in your life. Asking is a powerful way to navigate life.

Say:
I can ask for what my heart desires.

Never Ask "Why"

No matter how you ask, whether on your knees in tears or contemplating life in the shower, your effort to engage with this powerful presence is building and strengthening your relationship. But there are ways to be more effective and empowering in your asking.

First of all, ask the question that you want answered. Think of your higher power as the most powerful search engine on the planet, far more capable than Google. When you pose a question, the universe responds with answers that "match" the question. For example, if you ask the question "Why does this always happen to me?" the answers that are a match for the question will help you see why that thing always happens to you. But what you really want to know is *how* to move beyond the pattern.

As we've already seen, a more effective and empowering way to ask is to form your questions using *how, what, who,* or *where*. Here are examples of how these words can help you design a question that takes you where you want to go:

- **HOW:** *How can I move beyond this stuck place? How can I be what I desire? How must I change and grow to have what I desire?* It is important that *how* is asked with openness, expectancy, and curiosity. These inner states access your thriving Self. Doubt, anger, or resentment from your surviving self mindset limits your ability to change. If you are not sure how to ask *how* in an open, expectant, and curious way, at least ask the question while maintaining a smile on your face. A smile creates an internal openness. This open feeling is the energy you want when asking an effective and empowering question (EEQ)—no matter which of these four words you use.
- **WHAT:** *What must I do to have what I desire? What must happen for me to have what I desire? What must I learn? What must I let go of to have what I desire?*
- **WHO:** *Who must I become to have what I desire? Who are my teachers, champions, and mentors? Who are the members of my winning team? Who am I?*

- **WHERE:** *Where must I place my attention to manifest my dreams and desires?*

The role of the opening word of your questions is to help you be receptive to answers that are a match for your desire.

It takes practice to ask and then let go of the request and any doubt surrounding it. It takes maturity to understand and trust that some asks need setup time or an incubation period to manifest. The ask belongs to us, but the details of the delivery process belong to the same force that successfully governs the intricate, harmonious balance of the universe.

Not an ATM

Let's acknowledge that the great force is not an ATM created to service humankind. In life, if our interactions are centered around what another person can give us or do for us, the relationship is transactional and lacks true intimacy. Asking for assistance from our higher power can and should include asking for material things; having physical needs met is important. However, a relationship with the universe offers us the opportunity to cultivate a relationship where we feel safe and purposeful regardless of the material things we hope for.

There's a spiritual adage that says, *Don't be so focused on getting a Rolls Royce that you miss the Lear Jet the universe has for you.* When you ask with a fixed result in mind, you are asking for that Rolls Royce. But the answer that fulfills your heart might live outside your expectations. Ask from the energy of your thriving Self. Put your ask out to the universe. Imagine that your asks are seeds dropped into the soil of your higher power. Then leave room for results that stretch beyond your imagination.

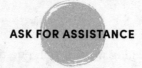

ASK FOR ASSISTANCE

A Revolutionary Act
Turn asking into a daily habit of acknowledging and
consciously striving to connect with your unseen force.

Inner Fitness Opportunity
Build a personal relationship with your higher power.

EEQ (Effective and Empowering Question)
Ask aloud:
How can I move out of my own way and
connect to something greater?

You Are More

—

I embrace the idea that I am more than any challenge I face.

THIS PRACTICE INVITES YOU TO REIMAGINE HOW YOU view yourself and appreciate the formidable power inside you.

The Starting Point

You are more than the thoughts that harass you, the secrets you keep, the hurt you've sustained, and the regrets, doubts, and insecurities you carry. You are more than your paycheck and debts, bad relationships, unfulfilling job, and life's daily demands.

I don't say this to make you feel good. It is the truth about you and everyone. However, if this concept feels good, great! That means you are open to its possibility.

We all want to be David and stand victorious before our Goliath challenge. Practice 3—*I embrace the idea that I am more than any challenge I face*—helps disrupt the negative tendencies of the surviving self and broadens our idea of ourselves and what's possible.

Like the universe, your infinite SELF is capable of always expanding and revealing new possibilities. Like in the Dream of Self, on page 41, your infinite SELF can step in, wrap its arms around you, and transform the hurt and disbelief of the surviving self. Remember that scientific research tells us that the brain is capable of change throughout our entire lives. This means we all have the inner power to address our challenges and make our lives feel better. No matter the problem, more freedom and joy are possible.

Embrace the Idea

The definition of *embrace* is to consider, think about, or support an idea. Practice 3—*I embrace the idea that I am more than any challenge I face*—encourages you to consider that there is a part of your essence that is connected to the greater force behind life. This part is unaffected by life's changing external circumstances and is known by many names.

Imagine listing every challenge or accomplishment that has or could ever confront you and saying about each one: *I am more than this [my great marriage, kids, success, and all the opposites of these].*

This mindset leaves room for a direct relationship with your higher power and distinguishes between the **infinite** part of you and the life challenges or circumstances you encounter. This distinction is crucial. Though the body and mind may experience challenges and human suffering, the infinite in you observes life, unaffected by life's changing nature. By being curious about the infinite, you can learn to see your circumstances through new eyes and discover less fearful and reactionary ways to experience your life.

A Not-So-Random Story About Acting

One of the best scenes of my career was left on the cutting room floor. I love acting. Getting to the truth of a character is one of my great joys. I've been fortunate to play a number of characters whose humanity came through me in a way that took my breath away. One such favorite moment was in an acting class when I was playing Lady Macbeth opposite Benicio del Toro. The life of Lady Macbeth moved through me in that scene in a way that had never happened before. Lady Macbeth moved me aside and came to life in my body. I willingly surrendered.

Another such opportunity to surrender to a character occurred during the writing of this book.

A wonderful director reached out to me to play a character I had never portrayed. I said "yes," first to the character, and then to my director friend. The character was a woman forced to carry the grief of decades of injustice.

I wanted to be her voice.

The night that we shot the scene in Texas, the character's life and pain rose in me during every take. I felt her say, "Excuse me, Tina Lifford, I need space," as she moved me to the side. At the end of the night, an executive producer shared that the producer's tent was quiet with awe after each take of the scene. One person characterized the scene as sublime. The lead actor and I had stepped into a historical reality, and we both let the moment happen.

Months later, after going through the postproduction process (where editing and a million other tweaks happen before the finished product is ready for public viewing), the director regretfully informed me that the riveting scene had been cut. She had no explanation why. She said something about a rewrite.

My response to this "heads-up" surprised me. I found myself unattached to the scene. I didn't feel loss, nor slight. How could I? I had experienced something "sublime." I had been a conduit for another's life and had touched lives in the process—and had been paid respectfully. It's not that I was above feelings like sadness or disappointment. These feelings are a part of the human experience. However, we are more than the thoughts and feelings we experience. In this case, I was not attached to being in or out of the production—neither defined me.

This response was Practice 3—*I embrace the idea that I am more than any challenge I face*—in action. I was more than a great performance and the choices, needs, and acts of others. I didn't need the film to prove my existence or impact. Everyone involved knew. The character lived. She had her say. The deleted scene went into my favorite bucket: Life is bumping into life, creating more life. As these circumstances bumped into my life, I expanded and became more of my thriving Self and infinite SELF. The circumstances didn't diminish me; they confirmed my expanding sense of Self, which I have been forging for decades.

Identification

When we attach our sense of Self to a persona—actor, mate, parent, rich, poor, powerful, insignificant, healthy, well, acceptable, or not good enough—we tell ourselves, *This is who I am.* The **surviving self's** role is to protect and reinforce our sense of ourselves, whether that sense empowers or diminishes us.

Whichever way we see ourselves, the surviving self will seek to hold on to and confirm this persona to the world. Putting our sense of Self in the hands of the surviving self is perilous. If I think a role defines me, then every role and acting experience has the power to give me a sense of Self or crush my sense of Self. Practice 3—*I embrace the idea that I am more than any challenge I face*—teaches me to trust that I am innately whole. No matter the challenge or circumstances before me, or how I or others see me, this practice reminds me I am more.

Vigilance is necessary. Without it, the surviving self's tendency to be defined by external factors, to take life personally, or to desperately try to be seen and approved of by the world overwhelms our sense of Self and disconnects us from our authentic thriving Self. The ability to shift our perspective and stay connected to an empowered sense of Self is the primary benefit of inner fitness. Practice 3—*I embrace the idea that I am more than any challenge I face*—helps us expand our definition of Self and break the identification with our personas.

Choose the Self

Shifting from habits of overwhelm, insecurity, and self-doubt to feeling like you are more than any challenge you face can feel like an unrealistic and unachievable leap. But leaping is not how you learn to believe you are more than any challenge you face.

Instead of leaping, always start by getting curious. Great EEQs—effective and empowering questions—for this are *What does this practice mean? How do I embrace the idea that I am more than any challenge I face? How can I move through this challenge? What are the thoughts, feelings, beliefs, and actions that will help me through this challenge?*

These EEQs provide the roadmap to lead you to the other side. This is the power of an EEQ. It penetrates doubt with vision, makes room for support, and helps you meet the challenge with the expectation of coming out on the other side whole and more of your Self. How you see yourself and respond during a challenge dictates its impact on your life.

By working with the Three Selves—the surviving self, thriving Self, and infinite SELF—you discover you are more than a weak and at-risk human being defined by external things and circumstances. Your essence is creative, resilient, and empowered to choose.

Your sense of hope or possibility can move mountains. You are whole, worthy, and powerful despite the problems and events you encounter. You can shift your focus away from the habit of allowing external things and situations to define you, and get curious about your innate value.

Ask:
What does it mean that I have undeniable innate value?

You Belong to the Universe

I have my family's receding hairline, my father's wit and left-hand tremor, my mother's smile and personality. When you see me with my family, the similarities in appearance and behavior are undeniable. I am certain you can name five traits you've gotten from your family and the environment in which you grew up.

However, to move through life and its challenges with a thriving mindset we must look beyond familial similarities to see our true nature and origin. You are not just the offspring of your human parents. Long before your parents got together and gave birth to you, there were billions or trillions of tiny adjustments in the universe preparing for you to enter life as a human being. The odds of being born human are 1 in 400,000,000,000,000. Your parents are a huge contributing factor to your birth, but they are neither the beginning of you nor the full story of who you are. You belong to the universe.

You are a mini version of the nature of the universe. Seeing your starting place as rooted in the universe and not just in your body allows your idea of Self to expand and allows you to bring more of your universal identity to any challenge you face. This is not about having faith, but rather, having inborn purpose. Once we know we have an innate purpose, we can stop allowing our hurtful histories to lie to us about our worth.

Ask:

How can I embody more of the nature of the universe in my
daily living?

A Thought to Ponder

What traits are instilled in every human being by the universe? The
scientific theory called the Big Bang tells us that the universe began
as a small dot that then exploded and expanded infinitely. Everything we know and all the questions that science has yet to discover
were inside that tiny dot. That cosmic explosion unleashed the unfolding universe that keeps expanding.

As the universe expands, more is revealed and known. When
gas, dust, and gravity came together in a particular way, our sun was
born. When the Earth bumped into a small planet, the moon was
created from the debris. Black holes are created from an extraordinary concentration of stress between energy and mass.

These examples show us one of the most profound statements
about the universe: The universe is a creative medium that constantly creates. Within it, things collide and new things are created. The universe takes the colliding in stride. It creates, resiliently
adapts, re-creates, and tirelessly advances.

If **life is always bumping into life**, then the best strategy for
thriving is to develop the ability to thrive no matter how life bumps
into you. The ability not to take life personally becomes a superpower. Effective and empowering questions you can ask are: *What
characteristics do I share with the universe?* and *How do I live life always advancing?* and *How do I learn not to take life personally?*

Mulling over such statements invests time with the higher
range of your Self and reminds you not to take life personally. Add
a thriving mindset to the statement, and you get this: *Life is bumping into life, creating more life, so how can I use this moment to thrive?*

This mindset opens you to thinking about what's possible and steers your thinking toward **solving problems instead of surviving problems**. Instead of being stuck in circumstances, you are open to best-case scenarios. This approach employs thriving characteristics like hope, imagination, vision, a sense of possibility, and openness to growth.

Working from the thriving mindset doesn't magically resolve difficult circumstances. But it allows you to navigate the circumstances with less stress, to be more aligned with your Self, and then to work intentionally. You can then meet your circumstances in a way that helps you grow instead of being bullied by circumstances into a corner where you feel powerless.

Say:

I am more than I know or give my Self credit for.

Ask:

How can I discover the more that lives within me?

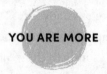

YOU ARE MORE

A Revolutionary Act

In the face of every challenge, setback, insecurity, or triggered response, say aloud to your Self, without any judgment, "I am more powerful than these circumstances," and then **EFFORT** (**E**xtracting **F**reedom **F**rom **O**ur **R**estricted **T**hinking) to lead with a thriving Self mindset.

Inner Fitness Opportunity

Teach yourself to address your issues and circumstances without being identified by them. When life bumps into you, remind your Self that you are more than the issues and circumstances before you. Use challenges as opportunities to grow.

EEQ (Effective and Empowering Question)

Ask aloud:

How can I experience life without being attached to a persona?

You Can Transform

———

*I look for and work to transform the beliefs, patterns,
and judgments I practice that limit my life.*

THIS PRACTICE CREATES AN EMPOWERED RELATIONSHIP
with things that disturb your peace.

Seeing What Is in Plain Sight

The life you want is always waiting for you. Even when you don't
know what you want to do, or how to move forward, a part of you
knows you want to feel better. Knowing you want to feel better is a
great starting place. It can be your roadmap to happiness and a more
fulfilling relationship with your Self.

We can't get to the life we want without first acknowledging the
things we don't want. If we want better relationships—for instance,
I want to feel safe and valued—we must acknowledge that our current relationships are unsatisfying and then go one step further and
identify the scenarios and experiences that represent what we no
longer want: *I want to feel safe and valued . . . but I feel attacked and
judged.* Or *I want to live with more peace, but I find myself often arguing and plotting war in my head.* Noticing that your life doesn't feel
good is an important step.

Acknowledging where we are in our lives can be challenging because it has been ingrained in our psyches that we should live performative lives and pretend we're happy. We dress up the outside self and hide the inner Self. On the outside our lives can appear to an observer to be almost perfect, while inside, we struggle with a discomforting or painful reality. Aligning our inner Self and outer projection creates an authentic Self, and in that Self there is room to thrive. Practice 4—*I look for and work to transform the beliefs, patterns, and judgments I practice that limit my life*—supports becoming aligned with your Self.

When I teach this practice in my workshop, inevitably, there are people who say they don't have patterns and find the practice assumptive. I appreciate their indignation. Their rejection of the assumption that they have patterns allows me to be curious and ask them questions. One woman felt my wording judged her and made assumptions about her without any personal knowledge of her. Compassionately, I asked whether this workshop was the first time she felt judged in this way. She shot back, "No, this has been happening my entire life!" The room was completely silent for a few beats. Then the woman and the entire room laughed. It took a moment for the woman to realize that if she's been reacting the same way for her entire life, *that's a pattern*. It takes a minute for us to see ourselves clearly sometimes.

Every human being has unconscious beliefs, patterns, and judgments that limit their lives. Research shows that the brain likes patterns. Habituating behavior offers a sense of certainty that the reptilian brain—the surviving self—seeks. The surviving self likes to travel roads it already knows because familiarity feels safe. Even if the same ol' road creates stress, the stress is familiar stress, and to the survival-focused brain, that's comforting.

Looking for the unseen beliefs, patterns, and judgments that limit our lives takes **EFFORT** (Extracting Freedom From Our

Restricted Thinking) to circumvent the brain's preference for the familiar. But uncovering patterns isn't as difficult as you might think; often, patterns hide in plain sight. Acknowledging them brings power into our lives.

Say:
To know my Self I have to look for my Self.

Where to Look

There is a fast, reliable way to see our beliefs, patterns, and judgments: Look at what challenges you or causes you to be upset or in pain. Right there will be your roadmap to freedom. When you discover what makes you feel insecure, unhappy, or lost—or whatever else is painful for you—you uncover three critical insights: (1) where you are, (2) where you want to be, and (3) how you want to feel. This information can become your guide. But so many people avoid looking at unhappiness. We walk around it and steer clear—and therefore delay feeling good.

We have been taught to be afraid of difficulty and to avoid painful emotions at all costs. But pain and challenges can help you thrive if used as a roadmap. Instead of seeing a difficult challenge as a problem, shift your thinking and allow it to highlight the part of you or your life in need of growth.

If you discover that you habitually react to life with fear, you can begin to use fearful moments consciously. By asking yourself a question like "What must I do to stop defaulting to fear so quickly?" your curiosity changes your relationship with the fear. Instead of running from fear, you are now courageously standing in front of it open and curious.

This vantage point makes room for ideas and answers that have not been accessible because of your previous avoidance or fear. Being curious helps you think better because curiosity flows from the thriving Self, which means you feel calmer and less fearful. The fear doesn't disappear immediately—rewiring our thinking takes time—but with every tiny adjustment, you are strengthened. You are less intimidated and more centered on yourself and what is possible for your life. You begin to feel you can stand up to old fear and win. Your habit of defaulting to fear begins to feel changeable and, therefore, less overwhelming.

For years I had no idea I buried my emotions. My "never let them see you sweat" game face was impenetrable. As I began to look for my authentic Self, I discovered a well of emotions. In that deep well were years of unresolved moments I had stuffed down instead of acknowledging and addressing them. As I acknowledged these emotions, I sometimes cried stored tears I didn't know I had. But more often, I experienced tears of joy and relief as I began to feel a new kind of safety: safety with myself inside myself. This felt like a new kind of freedom.

When we know where we are, we can better navigate away from there. We may have to cross choppy waters, but when the end goal is more peace and joy and access to our whole Self, experiencing dis-comfort in the journey is a small price to pay. The pain of rebirthing yourself can be as intense as the worst labor pains during childbirth. But that pain is overshadowed by the joy of you **thriving**—being resilient and authentic, and feeling full of possibilities.

Practice 4—*I look for and work to transform the beliefs, patterns, and judgments I practice that limit my life*—offers an almost step-by-step process for inviting more peace, joy, and Self into your life.

Three Powerful Words

Activating the first three words of this practice, *I look for*, will revolu-tionize how you engage with yourself and life. *I look for* is an action.

It is the EFFORT that turns difficulty and sadness into an opportunity for greater freedom and growth. If the premise is that *we are bigger than any challenge we face and capable of thriving no matter our circumstances*, then the effective and empowering question (EEQ) to ask is *How can I use these circumstances to thrive?* Every time you get curious, two powerful things happen. First, curiosity moves you to a higher consciousness because it engages the brain's frontal lobe, where the ability to think objectively and make nonreactive decisions is accessed. This part of the brain is where thriving lives. Characteristics such as hope, creative thinking, and envisioning new ideas and possibilities begin here. Second, when you are in this higher range of thinking, you can objectively observe yourself, notice your behavior, and interrupt unsupportive habits by identifying them and employing tools to turn them into supportive habits.

Look at Your Self

My client wanted a better relationship with her three teenage girls. Whenever she extended herself to them and attempted to ask how they were feeling, she felt they brushed her off. Each daughter would respond with a quick one-word answer: "Fine."

My client realized this one-word response was a pattern in her household. As she explored this pattern, two unconscious behaviors surfaced. First, she discovered that she was uncomfortable with feelings and often avoided them. She feared landing in an emotionally uncomfortable conversation that she couldn't navigate. So rather than feel impotent, she avoided feelings and emotional conversations. Second, my client realized that when she asked her girls, or anyone, "How are you feeling?" unconsciously, she *hoped* they would say "fine." "Fine" allowed her the satisfaction of seeming to show up as a concerned and loving mom but still steer clear of deeper emotions.

My client's desire to be a good mom instigated her engagement with Practice 4—*I look for and work to transform the beliefs, patterns, and judgments I practice that limit my life.* Her discomfort with her inauthentic behavior made her yearn to be more authentic and opened her to investing effort to be more present and engaging.

Once this client was willing to objectively *look at her beliefs, patterns, and judgments,* she was on the road to transformation and freedom. She became more honest with herself, and her family began to have more honest and meaningful conversations.

Say:
What I can see I can change.

Look to See

Often our unhelpful behaviors are unconscious, or so ingrained they are automatic. The only way to see behaviors that are on autopilot is to assume that below the surface of feeling unhappy, aimless, purposeless, unsettled, unvalued, unresolved, undecided, wandering, or unrooted is a belief, pattern, or judgment waiting to be seen. Don't be afraid to be curious. Lead with: *I embrace the idea that I am more than any challenge I face.* Realize it's okay to be afraid. Examining your fears is how you dismantle them and build inner fitness. With this mindset, Practice 4—*I look for and work to transform the beliefs, patterns, and judgments I practice that limit my life*—becomes an intention. In essence, you say to yourself, *Because I desire to thrive in my life, I set the intention to look for the thoughts, feelings, beliefs, actions, and reactions that limit me, and put EFFORT toward change.* Setting an intention is powerful because it sends a message that resonates with your heart and reaches your subconscious mind.

Once you set the intention *to look for,* almost magically you will begin to see previously unconscious behavior. Like the phenomenon of buying a car and suddenly seeing that car everywhere, setting an intention opens your eyes and allows you to see the kind of EFFORT needed to achieve new possibilities.

From this point forward, allow yourself to see opportunities in pain and difficulty instead of running from them. Seeing where you are and catching sight of your unconscious and limiting behavior is cause for celebration and a sigh of relief; when you know where you are, you can set your own journey. Making new choices is the work required to go from **surviving** to **thriving** throughout our entire lives.

A Where-to-Look Laundry List

It is impossible to create a list of all the places we can look to discover the beliefs, patterns, and judgments we practice that limit our lives. Each of us is unique in the ways tiny moments get under our skin and how we respond. But we all are human, and every human being has unconscious beliefs and blind spots. You can use the following list of common blind spots to give you an idea of where you might look to catch sight of your unconscious behavior.

- You always say "yes" or "no" first.
- You support others at the expense of neglecting or overlooking your Self.
- You feel angry or resentful when people don't behave as you expect.
- You begrudge the success, attractiveness, or intelligence of others.
- You feel aimless, purposeless, unsettled, unvalued, unresolved, undecided, wandering, or unrooted.
- You have areas where you behave with a lack of empathy and with a sense of entitlement, contempt, or arrogance.

- You prove yourself to others by manipulating, blaming, attacking, or judging.
- You second-guess yourself and doubt that others know what they are doing.
- You blame fear, lack of money, or circumstances for your inaction.
- You need to be in control.
- You let others run your life.
- You have a fraught relationship with your weight.
- You need to be angry to prove to the world how unfairly treated and hurt you have been.
- You prove your worth through your children, marriage, money, or other things outside of your Self.
- You expect to be rescued or taken care of.
- You need to rescue others and have answers for their lives.
- You think you are better than someone or that someone is better than you.
- You avoid difficult emotions by shopping, eating, having sex, drinking, or using drugs.

To thrive, adopt the habit of asking these two simple questions: *Is this a pattern in my life?* and *What belief or judgment against myself lives underneath this behavior?* You don't have to come up with the answers to these questions. Your EFFORT is to (1) ask the question, (2) ask for assistance (Practice 2) in catching sight of answers, and (3) have *I look for and work to transform the beliefs, patterns, and judgments I practice that limit my life* in the back of your mind all the time.

Now, with this internal insight and intention, people, circumstances, and realizations will surface to help you rise to new internal habits and heights.

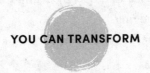

YOU CAN TRANSFORM

A Revolutionary Act
Set the intention to acknowledge pain and discomfort
rather than avoiding or running from them and
be curious about the growth they offer.

Inner Fitness Opportunity
Consciously use your fear to gain freedom from it.

EEQ (Effective and Empowering Question)
Ask aloud:
What is the starting place for transforming an old habit?

PRACTICE 5

You Can Choose

———

I can choose a Self-empowering response in any situation.

T HIS PRACTICE AFFIRMS YOUR POWER TO CHOOSE SELF-
care in any situation, including difficult moments when there
appears to be no choice.

24/7/365 You Have Choices

Housed within you is the inextinguishable power to choose what
is best for you, given your circumstances. Whether you are backed
into a corner or are feeling disrespected, abused, scared, anxious,
overwhelmed, lost, or depressed, your ability to choose how you
respond to your situation is a power that no one can take from you.
Being in a healthy, committed relationship with yourself that honors your Self is a superpower.

Before we are in a relationship or encounter other people, circumstances, or situations, we must first be aware that *we are in a
relationship with our Self.* Moment to moment, we are in an intimate
relationship with our thoughts, feelings, beliefs, actions, and reactions that shape and color how we see ourselves and the world. How
we are with ourselves sets the tone for how we respond to others
and how we will likely react in challenging situations.

If you are easily overwhelmed when things don't go as planned, this tendency will likely dictate how you think and react in tough times. If you are critical and impatient with yourself when you make a mistake, you give those simple errors the power to criticize and punish you. And, to the degree you extend grace to your Self, you give your Self permission to learn from mistakes and try again. You empower your emotions to be your friends or foes.

No matter how reactive you have been **up until now, from this point forward,** you can learn to be in ownership of yourself. Turning Practice 5—*I can choose a Self-empowering response in any situation*—into a skill makes you confident of your ability to navigate whatever life brings.

Say:
No matter how reactive I've been up until now, from this point forward, I can learn to make Self-empowering choices in any situation.

Disbelief

If you're shaking your head, thinking it is impossible to choose a Self-empowering response to some situations, I understand your response. In our 14 Practices workshop this practice always causes heads to shake and doubt to arise.

Here are the most passionate and sometimes tearful comments that follow a shaking head:

- *How can you say you can choose a Self-empowering response regarding sexual assault, especially when you are too young to know what's happening and your abuser threatens you?*
- *I wish I could have chosen a Self-empowering response when my mother died, but everything collapsed into nothingness, including me.*

- *The prison system works overtime to prove to you how powerless you are.*

Yes, scenarios like these are daunting. Yet millions of people have weathered such circumstances. So, the question to ask is how these people survived their circumstances. The better question is *How did they **thrive** beyond their circumstances?* What Self-empowering response did they choose?

A Self-Empowering Response

A friend was raped when she was in high school. I find few situations more heinous and abusive than the willful exercise of power over another that disregards their personhood and innate right to thrive. So, I was in awe of the response she chose that helped her hang on to herself during this criminal act: She had the very clear intention that even though the brute on top of her might take her body, she would not let him take her hopes and dreams and sense of Self. She was determined to hang on to her heart and soul, and she did. It took decades for her to process her sexual abuse fully, but she managed while cherishing her Self. She is proud of her response and herself.

Her heroic and revolutionary act was to distinguish between what was happening to her body and the essence of her—her infinite SELF. That Self-empowering choice enabled her to choose to tolerate her situation and simultaneously have a vision of her Self thriving on the other side. Though she had experienced something horrific, she had a plan for thriving. **Her choice made her present to the reality of her circumstances without making them part of her identity and becoming a victim.**

You choose a Self-empowering response any time you decide not to let a situation or moment become your final story. Regardless of the circumstances, you can fight to hold on to, love, and honor your Self by having a vision of your future, despite your inability to impact or change your current external situation.

In difficult circumstances, resiliency is forged by maintaining a sense that better days are ahead and envisioning your life beyond the present circumstances. No matter the scenario, when you focus on what you can create going forward rather than what's been taken or destroyed, you access the thriving Self and infinite SELF within you, which are creative and resilient, and empower you to choose how you respond to your situation.

Say:

The infinite SELF within me is more powerful than my external circumstances.

It's Never Too Late

Years ago, my disbelief in the idea that I could *choose a Self-empowering response in any situation* had me also shaking my head. The words sounded great, but implementing them seemed impossible, especially standing in my power when confronted by mean-spirited people.

There's no mystery as to why I used to feel overwhelmed by mean people. I grew up with cousins who were extremely mean-spirited during our youth, even though I love them today. They picked on me because I was different. I didn't care about the things most kids cared about. I was happy playing by myself and didn't try to hang out with them and their friends, nor did I admire that they had a lot of boyfriends.

But they were my cousins, and our being family meant something to me.

Nonetheless, spending time with them often reduced me to tears. They would seek to torment me by ignoring me or calling me names. They would laugh at me and call me a prude or Miss Goody Two-Shoes. They talked poorly about my mother to my face to get under my skin. I never felt I had the right words to fight them with. It was impossible to be myself with them. So, I was happy when my family moved three thousand miles away from my hometown of Evanston, Illinois, when I was thirteen.

But the pattern of feeling overwhelmed and sometimes frozen in place by meanness still lived within me. Until, in the 1990s, a neighbor unwittingly helped me rewrite my story and change my relationship to mean girls. This neighbor would be hot and cold with me and say mean things in a gaslighting way, sometimes being nasty and then pretending it was all a joke. I accepted this behavior several times. But each time I walked away from her, my stomach and heart felt out of sorts. I felt like I had with my cousins. And I didn't like it.

One day my neighbor was at my apartment and lobbed a cloaked verbal jab my way. I stared at her, counting to ten silently to connect with my Self. Then with kindness in my heart, I said, "I don't know why you make a point of being mean. I like you. But my friends don't treat me this way. If this is how you will be my friend, I can't have you in my life."

I don't know where those words came from. But they flowed from me effortlessly. She apologized and left my apartment soon after. When the door closed behind her, I felt brand-new. Something significant had changed. I came to realize that the encounter with my neighbor had allowed me to honor my Self. I had done nothing to this woman, and there was no reason to subject myself to such treatment. I knew I was not the cause of whatever drove her to behave that way. I had set a boundary and used my voice to support my inner Self. These were insights that I hadn't yet developed with my cousins back in Evanston. By addressing my neighbor, I sent a message of Self-honoring and Self-care to the deepest part of myself. The neglected parts and hurtful memories soaked that message up. I discovered I could choose how I wanted to be treated. I never worked at a friendship with that neighbor again.

When we choose to honor our Self, that choice always empowers. It doesn't matter how the situation turns out. The most important work—honoring your Self—is done.

Wicked or heart-wrenching circumstances like rape or death are more horrific in detail, and their pain is more evident and specific, than conflicts with cousins or a neighbor. But underneath our obvious suffering is the added pain of how we think about ourselves and treat ourselves because of the circumstances. This pain makes any situation worse. When we think we don't matter or see ourselves as less-than, not worthy, or any version of unacceptable or a failure, this causes our deepest suffering. The journey ahead is to know we matter and to replace our old default thinking with an authentic default to our thriving Self.

Say:

When I say "yes" to my Self, it is easier to set boundaries with others.

A Not-So-Random Story About Honoring the Self

During the COVID pandemic a beautiful woman, who was racked with pain, entered the inner fitness community. She had been suffering for almost two years from the death of her younger sister. This first-time visitor shared that she wished she could have died to spare her sister's life. Her love for her sister was palpable, but her love for Self was not. She had lost her connection to herself. Her sense of her innate value and undeniable worth were missing. She wanted to find her Self.

The most hurtful choices we make are against our Self. The most gratifying, healing, and empowering choices always honor our Self. It is never too late to live by this golden rule: Give your inner Self the honor it deserves.

No Exceptions to the Rule

Of course, in a life-threatening moment, with adrenaline pumping through our veins, Practice 5—*I can choose a Self-empowering response in any situation*—will look different. If a bear chases you, run like hell! That is the Self-empowering response of the moment. Fight, flight, or freeze is the empowered response in the face of physical danger. Helping us survive physical danger is the role of the surviving self. The inner drive for survival will force us to default to the millions of years of survival instincts encoded in our surviving self for our safety. However, Practice 5 teaches that after the dust of a reactive moment settles, you can choose a Self-empowering response that supports you in moving forward.

You can choose how you frame any experience in your mind.

Choosing a Self-Empowering Response

A Self-empowering response is any response that helps you remember you are more than your circumstances. When doubt or overwhelm show up, this is when statements like **"God doesn't make junk"** and **"Life is bumping into life, creating more life"** become tools that help us experience life without turning circumstances against us.

Choosing a Self-empowering response means taking an action that helps you reach for higher ground and think from your thriving

Self. Your thriving Self dreams, stretches, and strives to live beyond your restrictive thinking and circumstances. Activating thriving Self characteristics moves the mind to a more open, creative, and empowered state.

My parents were the first place I saw this behavior modeled. Of course, when I was a child, I didn't know then what I was looking at and how wise my parents were.

In our house when I was growing up, there were often more needs than money. However, we lived happy, well-fed lives because of my parents' creative resourcefulness. When money was tight, breakfast food became dinner. My mother would serve pancakes and eggs, and my sisters, brother, and I would feel like it was a special family treat.

When our heat was turned off for a few days one winter in Chicago, because of a past-due bill, the entire family piled into bed together in socks and long-sleeved shirts and had fun telling stories. During the next few days, my father was collecting bottles, emptying piggy banks, and borrowing money—resourcefully making ends meet.

Resourcefulness is a thriving Self characteristic. It challenges daunting circumstances and turns experiences into adventures. To the world, we appeared poor, but that was never encoded into my psyche because my parents responded to life with creativity, resilience, resourcefulness, and fun. All are thriving Self characteristics.

Say:
I can choose how I frame any experience.

How to Choose

Whether standing up to bullies in real time or recovering from a more heinous event, ultimately, to feel whole, we must honor our relationship with Self by making Self-honoring choices. When we are internally aligned with our worth, external circumstances take a backseat to our commitment to Self. Persecution, imprisonment, physical abuse, and difficult people may impact our physical bodies, but when we prioritize our relationship with the Self, these external forces can't distort or rule the inner Self. This is how the likes of Jesus, Nelson Mandela, Martin Luther King Jr., Gandhi, Nazi camp survivor Viktor Frankl, and Pakistani education activist Malala Yousafzai weathered difficult (or unimaginable) circumstances yet emerged unbroken and connected to something greater—an inner calling, mission, and purpose.

The Self-empowering response they each chose was to accept their limitations, or those imposed upon them, and hold on to a vision of life as it could be, to hope, to a sense of possibility, and to their connection to something greater than their circumstances.

Holding on to something greater is how you do not surrender your mind and Self when you are embroiled in challenging circumstances. Remembering that a responsive universal force made you, courses through you, and supports you in choosing a Self-empowering response in any situation.

In my youth, I didn't know how to respond to my cousins in a Self-empowering way. I didn't realize I had undeniable innate worth. However, when I began to learn this truth and feel it inside, I saw the pattern of overwhelm that was caused by my cousins.

When I fall into surviving self behavior such as worry, doubt, fear, and judgment, or I am overly cautious and narrowly focused, I know these tendencies represent the surviving self. Seeing this, I pull out my thriving Self word graphic of characteristics (page 65) and employ **EFFORT** (Extracting Freedom From Our Restricted Thinking) to shift my thoughts and feelings. I choose three to five characteristics to turn into action regarding my situation and see how I can respond to my circumstances in new or fresh ways.

Our thoughts and feelings are partners. Where one is, we will find the other. Together they create our reality. Therefore, learning to *shift* how you think or feel becomes a skill worth building: Notice when the surviving self predominantly drives your thoughts and feelings and then shift to thriving Self qualities and act from there.

For example, when I find myself at a choice point, these are some Self-empowering responses I choose: I acknowledge where I am and how I feel, and I envision how I want to be and feel in the future. Each of these responses affirms that I matter to myself. Here are the steps I take:

1. I acknowledge where I am and how I feel, and envision how I want to be and feel in the future. Each of these choices says I matter to my Self.

2. Because I know I am connected to a force greater than me that loves me and responds to my heart, speaking out loud, I ask the universe, *How can I move beyond this negative rumination?* Speaking out loud to the universe puts me in an active relationship with my Self and higher power.

3. I acknowledge the totality of my situation—out loud, at least ten times, using an affirmation like this: *Even though I am caught thinking the worst-case scenario, I deeply and profoundly love and accept myself.*
   Other sample affirmations:
   - *Even though I feel abused, I ASK to deeply and profoundly love and accept myself.*
   - *Even though I made an unhealthy choice, I ASK to deeply and profoundly love and accept myself.*

4. I don't monitor or judge each moment-to-moment effort. Constant monitoring indicates that anxiety and doubt are leading my efforts.

There's magic in *Even though I . . .* phrasing because it allows you to be honest and present about where you are while actively honoring yourself with the desire to deeply and profoundly love and accept yourself.

When I catch myself engaged in negative rumination, I know my surviving self is running on automatic. I aim to shift from a survival mindset to a thriving mindset. Practice 5—*I can choose a Self-empowering response in any situation*—reminds me to shift from surviving to thriving thoughts.

You Get to Choose

The goal is to bring your thriving Self to every problem, taking with you a sense of hope, possibility, greater freedom, curiosity, adventure, resilience, and **I-can-ability** everywhere you go. This mindset is not blind faith. It is active cultivation of your mental and emotional environments so that you can be and honor your Self in those moments and bring more life, options, and possibilities to them.

Life won't always show up as pleasant and fair. But you get to choose to what degree you take life personally, the meaning you assign to any set of circumstances, and how you see your Self.

Say:

I get to choose how I treat myself.

I get to choose to believe I matter.

I get to choose new possibilities.

I get to choose to use fear courageously.

I get to choose to heal.

I get to choose thoughts that empower me.

I get to choose how I see others and how I experience being seen.

I get to choose to live each moment as though it is my last.

I get to choose what I believe.

I get to choose to ask for and then recognize support.

I get to choose to change my mind.

I get to choose forgiveness over regret.

I get to choose to say "yes" to life.

I get to choose how I pray.

I get to choose gratitude, appreciation, and growth.

I get to choose my reality.

I get to choose freedom and joy.

I get to choose again . . . and again . . . and again.

I get to choose!

I choose my Self.

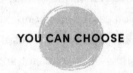

YOU CAN CHOOSE

A Revolutionary Act

Decide to take your power back from old choices by engaging in new behavior. However and at whatever age you lost connection with your Self, revisit in your mind the choice you made and envision what a Self-empowering choice might look like. Then, from this point forward, in similar scenarios, respond to such choices with your Self-empowering response.

Inner Fitness Opportunity

Rise to a higher level of Self-care and personal power.

EEQs (Effective and Empowering Questions)

Ask aloud:

How can I make a Self-empowering response despite being afraid?

What is a Self-empowering response that I can make
today regarding a past situation even if I am no
longer connected to the person or people who were
involved? (Asking the question is the crucial act.)

No More Self-Rejection

—

I make a list of ways I mistreat and reject
myself and begin to treat myself better.

T HIS PRACTICE LETS YOU OBJECTIVELY SEE YOUR RELA-
tionship with yourself and work to improve it.

A List Is Powerful

Everyone loves a good list. Grocery. Back to school. Things to do
today. Lists help you accomplish and manage the items on them.
But how many people make a list of things they admire and accept
about themselves to have a clear understanding of their strengths
so they can continue to move in a positive direction? Or rarer, how
many people are willing to make a list of ways they mistreat themselves so they can clearly see how they undermine themselves in
order to shift their behavior and thrive? These two lists have the
power to change your life for the better. They allow you to see where
you are in your relationship with your Self and give you a roadmap
for making this relationship the best it can be. Taking time to make
a list that helps you "see what needs to be seen" in your life, as stated
in the intention statement on page 14, reveals to you the untruths

and misperceptions you carry that obscure this truth: **You are capable.** You can flourish and thrive. You have inside you what you need to address your desires and challenges. Making a list of ways you mistreat and reject your Self is one of the most life-enhancing lists you will ever make. Practice 6—*I make a list of ways I mistreat and reject myself and begin to treat myself better*—helps you see your limiting beliefs and unkind behavior toward your Self so you can reject the behavior and embrace your whole Self.

Say:
Saying "I see you" to behavior that does not honor me is an act of Self-love.

No Need to Avoid This List

In our workshops, people fear acknowledging the ways they mistreat themselves because they think admitting to their behavior will make it more overwhelming and harder to live with. **When we run from ourselves—judge, distrust, or lack compassion for ourselves—that is Self-rejection.** Many people attempt to ignore their difficulties and pretend not to see the unpleasant parts of their lives.

But avoiding or hiding from problems is not productive. It, too, is a form of Self-rejection.

Hiding signals that we judge our challenging areas as unacceptable and doubt our ability to navigate them successfully. The message we subconsciously send to ourselves is: *This part of me is so unacceptable that I can't bear to look at it.* But this thought belongs to fear. It is not true. It is just a thought.

There's a school of thought that says the areas that cause us discomfort are the ones seeking healing attention.

Science Says

Many psychological theories and models suggest there is an aspect of the psyche that strives for healing, balance, and homeostasis. Homeostasis is the body's and mind's effort to seek internal stability. In some theories, Self-actualization—the drive toward fulfillment of one's potential and personal growth—represents an intrinsic desire to achieve wellbeing.

When you fear the discomfort of your history and your surviving self laments *I'm not as good, smart, capable, lovable as . . . I can't . . . I didn't have . . . I wasn't . . . I'm not . . . I don't . . .* there's a lie within this thinking that is trying to get your attention so you can dismantle it and move toward the truth. You are creative enough to design and redesign your life, resilient enough to weather any storm, empowered to choose and rechoose how you think about your life, mystically whole, and undeniably worthy. This truth supports creating an internal environment conducive to inner healing, balance, and homeostasis.

The thriving Self is always your doorway to this truth. It helps you regulate your thinking and return to a sense of your personal possibility and capability when your surviving self is caught in a triggered or reactionary state. This is why inner fitness emphasizes the need to maintain a strong thriving Self. It is the conduit between the tunnel vision of the surviving self and the truth and calm of the infinite SELF. The thriving Self stands in the gap, aware of the surviving self and the infinite SELF, and is committed to being the meeting place where healing, balance, and homeostasis can occur.

Let's revisit Thich Nhat Hanh's two analogies: he explains that it is impossible to have a "right" side without having a left. The right cannot be pulled or separated from the left. Cut the left side off, and another left takes its place. One creates the other. This makes the right and left one, not two.

Within our desires for freedom is a lack of freedom that makes the idea of freedom possible. *No mud, no lotus.*

Practice 6—*I make a list of ways I mistreat and reject myself and begin to treat myself better*—turns the list we make into the mud that makes the lotus. The thriving Self uses the laments of the surviving self to reveal the truth, and the truth sets us free. When the surviving self focuses on inadequacy, the thriving Self turns life over to the greater force and asks to feel capable, connected, and whole.

Say:

Every part of me is worthy and deserves my compassionate care.

A Not-So-Random Story About Self-Rejection

I have a brilliant client who wins at everything she does. She is a revered leader—thorough, thoughtful, consistent, and often considered a dream to work with. Her success is hard-won. She's gotten there by being overly prepared and vigilantly dotting her i's and crossing her t's. She has viewed her exactness as a superpower; however, her outer success came with an internal grind that kept her stressed and up at night, so she could look for and get ahead of every potential problem. She constantly picked at herself, demanding perfection. Unconsciously, she focused on proving her value instead of fulfilling her innate potential.

Growing up, her parents were demanding. She learned to reject the notion of herself and her talent as "enough." She always had to do more to prove her worth. No matter her long list of accomplishments, earned bonuses, or the pats on the back she received, she saw herself as unacceptable or not good enough.

Striving to be the best may seem admirable; however, inner fitness doesn't lead with external achievements. Self-acceptance, inner strength, and learning to be with your Self are the focus.

I asked my client whether she could achieve her desired success with less angst and more Self-love, grace, and ease. Her immediate answer was "No!" Followed by, "In business, you're only as good as the numbers." I rephrased my question and asked whether she would *like* to experience more grace and ease in her process. Her eyes filled with bewilderment. Then she said, "I've never even considered such a thought." She paused. "Grace and ease and being less hard on myself would be fantastic, but I don't see how that's possible with the sharks in my waters."

I suggested, as an exercise, she forget her external environment and focus only on how she is with herself. I asked her to list her key beliefs and what she tells herself privately. Here is her partial list:

- I believe that if I'm not perfect, I'm not valuable.
- I don't trust that things will work out for me because I've had to fight every step of the way.
- I'm terrified of being seen as less-than and discounted as irrelevant.
- I see mistakes as failures.
- I see myself as responsible when anything goes wrong and hate myself when they do.

The final question I asked her was "If your external world stayed the same and you changed your internal relationship with yourself, would that bring more grace and ease to your life?"

She paused again. "Yes. I'm super hard on myself."

We all have a bit of this client in us. Her expressions of Self-rejection—proving her worth, making unreasonable demands of herself, judging herself harshly, and rarely patting herself on the back—may not be yours, but the nature of the surviving self is to normalize our learned limiting behavior.

Ask:

How do I set my WHOLE Self free?

No More Self-Rejection

We are the universe in action. Each of us is connected to the intelligence that organizes the entire universe, wires the brain, and drives the systems that make life possible. With such power and potential inside, what prevents us from interacting with our creativity and potential with greater trust and eagerness?

The answer is that the surviving self has been in charge. Up until now, we were less familiar with the thriving and infinite aspects of SELF that expand us beyond the habits of the surviving self.

No one taught us not to take it personally when life bumps into us or to objectively sit in our observer's chair and say "I see you" to behavior that undermines our ability to thrive. We weren't taught to see ourselves as **innately creative, resilient, empowered to choose, whole, and worthy**; or to consciously use our thoughts, feelings, and beliefs as powerful positive tools; or to ask effective and empowering questions (EEQs). We didn't know that Self-awareness and the introspective, reflective abilities of the **thriving Self** could help us survive in new, life-enriching ways that expand us beyond the habits of the **surviving self**.

We had no idea that making a list of ways we mistreat and reject ourselves could be the pathway to **deeply and profoundly loving and accepting ourselves**.

Say:
Every challenge in my life can lead to freedom when I use it to thrive.

The Many Faces of Self-Rejection

You must look for and work to transform the beliefs, patterns, and judgments you practice that limit your life (Practice 4) to consciously support your "mud" transforming into flowers.

Identifying the obvious ways that you mistreat and reject your Self is easy. Here's a litmus test: You call yourself names like "stupid" or "idiot"; you call yourself a failure or you intentionally hit or physically hurt yourself; you harshly judge yourself and often default to feeling unworthy; or you regularly lead with "I can't," "I'm not," "I didn't have," "I wasn't," and "I don't" statements. For example: "I can't make that kind of money/have a good relationship/feel good about myself *because* . . ."

More subtle signs of mistreating your Self include characterizing your Self as weak and shameful, or telling your Self any story that limits your ability to thrive.

You might think labeling such behavior as abusive is dramatic and distasteful. I've had people argue that everyone judges themselves harshly or calls themselves names sometimes. And this is true. Such behavior is the nature of the surviving self—we all look for what's wrong and are sometimes intolerant of and impatient with ourselves and others. But acknowledging that this behavior is normal doesn't mean it is useful nor does it negate that it mistreats the Self. Therefore, interrupting the slightest acts of mistreatment is a habit worth cultivating.

If something is precious and you treat it as though it isn't, even for a second, you are mistreating its preciousness. You must see this and want to do this less and less.

When your ill-treatment leaves you feeling worse about your Self, or leads to walking away from your dreams or doubts about your capableness or ability to thrive, then that mistreatment rejects the idea of your Self as innately precious, worthy, and connected to a force greater than your small idea of Self.

Science Says

Self-rejection can lead to feelings of worthlessness and Self-loathing that elicit a pain response in the brain as impactful as physical pain. The results of Self-rejection include shame, guilt, and sadness. It can impair thinking, decision-making, and problem-solving, and make it difficult to develop a positive Self-image.

Ill-treatment of your Self must be deemed unacceptable. As I say in *The Little Book of Big Lies*, "There is never, ever a justifiable reason to harshly judge [your] Self—not for any reason, under any circumstances. It is simply unacceptable."

Say:

My innate value deserves my love and support.
My biggest gift to my Self is to be compassionate with my Self
no matter the circumstances.

Extending love to your Self is good for your health. You must tell your Self you matter. Apologize to your Self for discounting, rejecting, and minimizing your value. You must hold your Self close, rock your Self, and whisper to your Self, *I am sorry you feel so hurt.* You must be patient like a mother is patient with a lost and flailing newborn who understands nothing and needs a caregiver to guide the way. You must be lighthearted, laugh, and say often, "Life is bumping into life, creating more life," and not take it personally.

Caring for your Self in loving ways and finding reasons to laugh often releases hormones that support creating an internal environment conducive to healing. Consciously engaging in these behaviors sends the message that we matter to the deepest part of us. This is how we learn to thrive.

Practice 6—*I make a list of ways I mistreat and reject myself and begin to treat myself better*—makes you more conscious of the unhealthy ways you interact with your Self and you can turn this awareness into loving guidance.

Say:

Up until now, I harshly judged my Self and focused on how I
was unacceptable to my Self and others, but from this point
forward, my behavior can change for the better.

From This Point Forward

Our mistreatment of Self is so ingrained that we often can't see it plainly; evidence of it lives in our Self-judgment and lack of joy.

When we see these signs, stepping in with a heartfelt Self-hug is a great first step.

When you can't see your blind spots yet feel unhappy with your Self, assume your surviving self is dictating this experience. Get curious. Be in a compassionate relationship with your Self. Ask your Self what you need and then let your Self voice your unspoken fears or sadness. Acknowledge your fears. But leave room for the spirit of Practice 3—*I embrace the idea that I am more than any challenge I face.* Aloud, tell your Self you're sorry for the pain you feel.

Ask:

What must I see and change to love and appreciate my Self?

Asking this question instigates a deeper, more supportive engagement with your Self.

Then climb into your observer's chair and objectively watch yourself through the next several days. Your intention to treat your Self better will help you see unconscious, unhealthy behaviors that need to change.

While seated in their observer's chair, many people in our workshops have had life-changing insights about their rejection or mistreatment of Self, such as:

- I reject my Self when I allow others to mistreat me.
- I reject my Self when I don't like looking at myself in the mirror.
- I reject my Self when I don't speak up out of fear.
- I reject my Self when I am confused and my ego won't ask questions.
- I reject my Self when I beg others to love me.
- I abuse my Self when I constantly rehash or relive the past.

- I reject my Self when I feel I have to get back at others.
- I reject my Self when I dim my light to fit in or to accommodate the discomfort of others.
- I abuse my Self when I act like I have the power to save others at the expense of my wellbeing.

Whatever you discover when sitting in your observer's chair, add it to your list of ways you mistreat and reject your Self, and then use the list as guidance to behave in the opposite way. For example, if you tend to reject your thriving Self by saying "no" to new experiences, start saying "yes," "maybe," or "I'll consider it." Then sincerely take time to consider engaging in the new experience.

Say:
My list is a roadmap for new behavior.

My Experience

I've had many aha moments sitting in my observer's chair. I most cherish the realization that I reject my infinite SELF whenever I act out of fear. I have realized that if everything is connected, thriving is defined as using every challenge to grow, and my growth is my ultimate purpose. I sabotage my growth and block fulfilling my purpose when I let fear stop me. Conversely, every time I challenge fear, I grow and reveal more of the infinite power and nature behind life, and I become a higher version of my Self.

Acting from fear says I am invested in the lie called failure. But how can failure be a real concept if I use it to grow into more of my Self? From this perspective, failure becomes irrelevant, and focusing on how a moment can help me grow becomes the win in any circumstance. If I am willing to grow, I win—even if the result looks like failure to others. With this mindset, I am always fulfilling my purpose.

If I indulge fear, I make people and circumstances more important than my potential and possibilities, and I diminish myself in the process. Every choice I've made from fear has limited my potential for growth.

New considerations and actions interrupt old patterns. That interruption is the **EFFORT** (**E**xtracting **F**reedom **F**rom **O**ur **R**estricted **T**hinking) it takes to build a new pattern or way of being your Self. Practice 6—*I make a list of ways I mistreat and reject myself and begin to treat myself better*—is the most valuable, life-enhancing list you can make if you want to thrive.

Say:
My list leads me to my liberation.

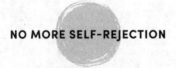

NO MORE SELF-REJECTION

A Revolutionary Act
Despite any fear or avoidance of this practice, make a list of at least three ways you mistreat or reject your Self. Then list behaviors that would take you in the opposite direction.

Inner Fitness Opportunity

Give your Self compassion and a goal.

EEQ (Effective and Empowering Question)

Ask aloud:

What must I realize to be in alignment with
my Self and love my Self more?

Make Peace

---

*I release all people and things from the
responsibility of making me happy.*

THIS PRACTICE HELPS YOU REALIZE THAT *YOU* ARE RE-
sponsible for *your* happiness and must learn to generate happiness from within your Self.

Breathe a Sigh of Relief

Never again do you have to wait for people and life to show up
a certain way for you to be happy. You can teach yourself to take
ownership of your joy. When you make other people and things responsible for your happiness, happiness becomes conditional: *When*
things between you and another person are good, *then* you can be
happy; *when* you get what you want from someone or acquire some
"thing" you think you need, *then* you can be happy. This *when I . . .
then I* approach gives the responsibility for your internal state to
others. This backward orientation negates your power to generate
happiness that isn't tied to a person or thing and renders you reactive rather than being the creator of your internal experience.

You can take charge of how you *experience* life and the meaning
you assign to events. You can remain standing when life bumps

into you. No matter how unpredictable life can be, you can forge a rock-solid inner state that isn't reliant on other people or things stepping in to make you happy. Practice 7—*I release all people and things from the responsibility of making me happy*—makes how you are with yourself the ultimate source of feeling good about yourself and life.

Say:
My happiness starts within me.

You Are Your Source

My sister Marty, who passed away in 2017, was the pretty one, inside and out. And fashionably petite. People would see her and fawn, "Well, aren't you a pretty little thing!" If they noticed me standing behind Marty's bright light, they would politely search my face and finally say something about my big eyes. From grade school far into womanhood, I was rarely noticed when standing next to most of the women in my life. The boys I had crushes on were interested in pretty girls, and then pretty women, like my sister. Between my mean cousins who bullied me and these regular negative messages about my beauty, I learned early that living a happy life would require me to figure out how to approve of and be happy with my Self.

It helped that I could entertain myself. There were no mean people in my imaginary world, and my beauty was a given, and unimportant. I wanted to do and see so many things—like, go to Africa, be an actress or a model, and learn stuff that mattered to me. In my early teens, I mostly wanted the freedom to be myself. I wanted to cartwheel to my friend's house, even if it wasn't the way most people traveled; stand on my head for as long as I wanted; think about things that pleased me; and ask a bazillion questions, even if it made me seem weird.

As I grew older, I wanted to use curse words because I liked the energy in them. The word *fuck* says so much, perfectly. I didn't want to feel pressured to live according to the beliefs, rules, and needs of adults or my friends. I wanted time to think about life and take a stab at living it on my terms. I didn't know it back then, but my soul wanted to trust in Practice 1—*I practice turning my life over to a power greater than me that loves me and responds to my heart.* I yearned to live this life making heart-aligned choices and navigating with faith. Practice 7—*I release all people and things from the responsibility of making me happy*—puts us in an active relationship with the infinite SELF at our core.

Say:
Everywhere I go, my whole Self goes with me.

Let Go

We are taught that our happiness comes from a chain of events: growing up, getting an education, getting a job, getting married, buying a house, and having kids. This path to happiness has been sold to us as tried and true for hundreds of years. Well, it is certainly tried. However, the true part isn't so true; it is not a recipe for happiness no matter how often it has been followed.

Happy moments abound. Your wedding day, a birthday, a promotion, a great movie, or a day at the park all deliver short-term happiness. But long-term happiness emerges from satisfaction with Self that you can pull from, even in difficult times. This happiness isn't a guarantee that comes with life. You can't give it to someone or receive it in exchange for anything.

Rather, it is an internal emotional tendency forged and strengthened through specific **EFFORT** (Extracting Freedom From Our Restricted Thinking): getting to know, understand, and accept yourself; acknowledging your likes and dislikes; acting in alignment with your Self; being accountable to your beliefs and needs; living with a positive sense of what is possible for your life; and compassionately working with yourself inside your Self during difficult emotional events. These choices are the fountain from which long-term happiness flows. Unhappiness—a disconnect from Self in the ways just mentioned—is guaranteed when you forgo this kind of EFFORT.

Happiness is a difficult state for anyone to achieve. The brain was designed to focus on survival above all else. Although the ability to thrive is innate, happiness is a cultivated state. Happiness can only live in our hearts to the degree that we manage the negativity bias of the surviving self. This is why inner fitness practices are necessary. The awareness and management of our thoughts, feelings, and beliefs is critical.

When we require others to be responsible for our happiness, we require them to have the capacity to figure out what will make us happy and manage our surviving self so that happiness can actually penetrate our surviving self habits. Whew! That's a lot of weight and work that will eventually disappoint you and the other person, adding frustration or stress to the relationship. Practice 7—*I release all people and things from the responsibility of making me happy*—strongly encourages us to release our expectation of people and things as our saviors or road to fulfilling our whole Self.

In one of my workshops, a community member chose to focus on Practice 7 for a week. In our Practice 7 deep dive, she shared this:

> I've always looked to others for happiness. The first time I read Practice 7—*I release all people and things from the responsibility of making me happy*—my mind exploded. I think my jaw dropped. I thought my husband, family, and friends were supposed to

bring me happiness. I can't tell you how often I blamed or resented them for my bad mood. I believed I would be happy if they just behaved in a different way. I saw *them* as the problem.

But the more time I spend practicing inner fitness, the more I realize my happiness is not their responsibility. I'm looking at my marriage in a different way. I didn't know if I wanted to stay married because my husband wasn't making me happy. But I finally realized my happiness wasn't his responsibility. I've expected him to achieve the impossible. So, as I'm doing these inner fitness deep dives and learning how to apply this to my life, I am experiencing more joy. I'm making myself happy through just learning who I am. And it's a good feeling.

Ask:
What does it take to be in charge of my happiness?

How to Build Your Happy
By **upgrading your knowledge of Self,** you upgrade your beliefs about who you are and what is possible in your life. This mindset fosters a kind of happiness that is less about people and things and more about YOU—your relationship with your Self and how you respond to life.

When you realize that you can choose a Self-empowering response in any situation (Practice 5), then **the actions of other people and difficult situations do not dictate your life. You take charge of your internal state,** and your Self-empowering responses lead. When your mate doesn't do what they promised, or you have financial issues, or you are feeling down, you can pause, **remember that you are the governor of your inner state.** Instead of blaming the external world, turn to your Self, **shift your mindset, examine your expectations,** and **choose a Self-empowering response.**

Releasing others from the responsibility of making you happy means you can always care for yourself by **being compassionate with yourself** in such moments, **without resenting others**. If your mate forgets to do something on the to-do list, if your boss isn't showing you the kind of appreciation you desire, or if you are suddenly overwhelmed by the demands of your kids or life, instead of blaming them or turning their behavior against yourself and feeling burdened, you can shrug your shoulders and say, "Life is lifing." Then, choose one or more of the 14 Practices or other tools in this book to turn challenges into personal growth.

This wellbeing mindset places you in a healthy relationship with your Self. From this mindset, people and things can add sparkle and value to your life without becoming your life.

Say:
I cultivate a joyful relationship with my Self and allow others to add sparkle and value.

Happiness Starts with You Not Things

You can spend years uncovering the wisdom packed in a transformational statement. This has been my experience with the mindset of Practice 7—*I release all people and things from the responsibility of making me happy.*

I remember as a teenager being crestfallen because someone didn't want to be my friend. My mother was at the kitchen sink rinsing green beans. She turned her head toward me and with a "that doesn't make any sense" tone said, "So, are you going to be unhappy for the rest of your life because somebody doesn't like you?" Mommy's tone and words together worked magic. The notion of being sad forever because "whoever" didn't like me did not make sense. Her question delivered the intended result. I let go of wanting anything from that girl.

Similarly, years later, when I was sixteen or seventeen, I was taught another memorable lesson about the power of Practice 7—*I release all people and things from the responsibility of making me happy.* I worked after school at a tool supply shop that employed both my father and mother. The owner, Don Lease, was a teddy bear of a man, with a big heart. He clearly liked the work ethic of our family. He owned a green flower-top Plymouth Barracuda that his wife rarely drove. Mr. Lease offered to sell the car to me on a payment structure I could afford. Beaming, I jumped at the opportunity. I loved the mod top, and the idea of being the responsible owner of a cool car made me proud.

Fewer than two months after I got the car, my sister was driving it and side-swiped a pole. I was beside myself and fighting mad at my sister. This time, my father's words taught me a slightly different version of the lesson my mother had taught me standing at the kitchen sink. Daddy said, "It's just a car." My parents were helping me see that neither people nor things should be the source of my happiness. They were making me ready for the reality that people and things come and go. If I hooked my happiness or sense of Self to external sources, I would have cause to worry and feel at risk regularly. **A life well-lived holds on to itself internally despite the ebb and flow around it.**

The notion of happiness being generated from the inside out resonated and made sense. Whenever I caught myself grinding on some thought that aimed to assign blame and responsibility to another person for how I was feeling, I would interrupt that thinking by shaking my head to shake free of my outward focus and blame. I became a pro at seeing when I was thinking of myself as a victim and heading down a path of blame. I learned to shake my head and say out loud, "It's only a thing." These words would give me distance from the habit of feeling wronged and allow me to reset my thinking.

What's Worth Giving Away

Things come in all shapes, sizes, and forms. Some of the crucial things we need to let go of aren't physical things at all. They might be the things we hold on to that block access to what we most desire.

I worked with this practice for more than a decade before a workshop participant took its wisdom to a different depth. She called herself a pre-worrier: On her days off, or when life was going well, she found herself worrying about something weeks down the road or things that didn't require any worry at the time. She shared examples of how she rushed to worry, including the memory of being four years old and worrying about whether her loving parents would return whenever they left the house. She spoke with such preoccupation with worrying, it was clear this habit was her way of navigating life. She believed that pre-worrying kept her prepared and safe from being blindsided by life. It was a light bulb moment for her to see her pre-worry as the "thing" she needed to release to experience the trust she ultimately desired.

We all have some experience that has become a "thing" in our lives. When we identify with that thing or issue, we begin to live with it like we have no other option, we give our power to that thing, and unknowingly, we limit our sense of Self and what's possible for our lives.

But what if thinking about our problems as our limitation is the "thing" we must let go of to make room for happiness? What if it is possible to be happy with yourself despite your so-called limitations? Might it be possible to recognize and live with this challenging human facet and still be whole, be capable, and have infinite possibilities?

It is difficult and counterintuitive to be okay with the thing that we find most challenging, shameful, embarrassing, and debilitating. But what if you could use this difficult part of your life for growth and that growth made more room for joy?

When we become curious about our ability to be happy and know joy despite our circumstances, the power of Practice 7—*I release all people and things from the responsibility of making me happy*—becomes more useful and usable.

Here's a short list of "things" you can set your intention to release:

- Suffering
- Feeling broken, less-than, or not good enough
- Self-judgment
- Anger
- Resentment
- Guilt

You can aim to use every challenge to love, accept, see, feel, and know your value. Transform your challenges into aha moments, a healing process, and a profound inner journey to Self-acceptance.

Imagine living a life that can accept and manage the challenges of being human and learn from them without letting them block happiness or rob you of your peace.

Say:
Every person, place, thing, and internal state I encounter can be used to forge the happiest me ever.

MAKE PEACE

A Revolutionary Act
Choose the most challenging experience of your life and
use it to forge rock-solid happiness with your Self.

Inner Fitness Opportunity
You get to smile and experience more positivity because
you use everything to grow into the best version of you
and expand your relationship with your inner Self.

EEQs (Effective and Empowering Questions)
Ask aloud:
How do I become connected enough with my Self that I give people
the grace to be themselves rather than who I NEED them to be?
How can I discover what I need to let go of and enjoy letting go?

Accept Your Self

———

I ask to profoundly accept my Self and believe in my value.

THIS PRACTICE HELPS YOU SKILLFULLY AND COMPASSION-ately work toward Self-acceptance.

You Have Innate Value

When the universe poured its life into you, your innate value was solidified. You were given a distinctive fingerprint and DNA that the universe responds to. You were born innately creative, resilient, empowered to choose, whole, and worthy. *Whole* means you have everything you need inside of you, and therefore, you have the power to change your life with how you think and behave. Your worthiness comes with your existence, instilled in you by a force that is greater than you, that created you, and that deems you innately good. These truths live at the core of you. The infinite SELF within you has never judged you nor left your side. Practice 8—*I ask to profoundly accept my Self and believe in my value*—teaches you to give your Self the acknowledgment you deserve and to remember that the deepest part of you never forgets that you matter.

Say (with your hands over your heart):
I matter. (Repeat three times.)

Imagine waking up daily with profound Self-acceptance, feeling equipped to address and skillfully navigate the most challenging aspects of your life, caring for your Self mentally and emotionally with love, and having deep trust in your ability to navigate any stress or difficulty before you.

With Practice 8—*I ask to profoundly accept my Self and believe in my value*—you are asking the universal force, which is greater than you, to help you see that you are more than your patterns, beliefs, feelings, and reactions. These are your circumstances and details. They are not you, nor do they represent or impact your value. You are more (Practice 3). Your value is in your existence.

Profoundly Accept Your Self

In our workshop deep dive into this practice, I ask participants to look up the definition of *profound*: (1) (of a state, quality, or emotion) very great or intense; (2) (of a person or statement) having or showing great knowledge or insight; (3) (of a subject or thought) demanding deep study or thought; (4) penetrating or entering deeply into subjects of thought or knowledge, having deep insight and understanding.

Next, I ask each person to write in their journal what *profound* means in the context of their Self-acceptance. Here are several answers:

- To accept my Self very deeply.
- To know myself deeply, accept my values, and know who I am.
- I am great.
- I accept even the things I don't like or am not proud of.

- I can't expect to be understood if I don't deeply understand and accept myself.
- I am in touch with what moves me.
- To understand why I do things or feel as I do.
- I can say "no" to people who don't feel safe.
- I don't have to believe the hurtful lies I've been told.
- I can be profoundly emotional and accept myself.
- I need to spend more time with myself.
- I can study myself like I study anything else that I want to be skilled at.
- I can deeply accept myself as a work in progress and let go of any shame.
- I can gain deep knowledge of my Self and my feelings by telling myself the truth.

Say:

Within my Self-acceptance, I discover the Self that knows I am enough.

Self-Appreciation vs. Self-Acceptance

Self-appreciation refers to recognizing and valuing what you do well, how far you've come, and celebrating your unique contributions to the world. **Self-acceptance** means embracing, without judgment, all of yourself, including your strengths, weaknesses, and mistakes, as well as the parts you might wish were different.

In the first version of the 14 Practices, Practice 8 was written with the word *appreciate*—*I ask to profoundly **appreciate** my Self and believe in my value*. However, in workshop or retreat settings, I saw a significant difference in the participants' experience when focusing on Self-appreciation rather than Self-acceptance.

Self-appreciation gave participants a joyous feeling. They loved acknowledging their uniqueness and positive qualities and basking in their glow. However, I discovered that some participants could not sustain their Self-appreciation postretreat; for many people, our Self-appreciation exercises were a way of ignoring what they didn't like and judged about themselves. They focused only on what they appreciated. When they returned to their postretreat lives, Self-judgment and Self-doubt would kick in and make sustaining their Self-appreciation difficult.

Self-Acceptance

Self-acceptance creates a profoundly intimate relationship with your Self.

It means acknowledging and embracing all aspects of ourselves, including our flaws and limitations; sober acknowledgment of all facets of ourselves is the path to knowing ourselves. Can you sit with yourself and tell your Self the truth without judging your Self and seeing yourself as unacceptable? It is this effort of extending loving compassion to ourselves instead of Self-judgment that turns Self-acceptance into an intimate act.

My Experience

I used to be incredibly judgmental. How we treat others is a strong indicator of how we treat ourselves. I didn't realize it then, but my quick judgment of everything and everybody was my unconscious strategy for feeling safe in the world. I believed if I could put something or someone in a box, I could better manage my fear of the unknown regarding that person and life, and be ready for whatever might happen. For example: If I placed you in my untrustworthy box, I acted like I knew who you were, and I projected my beliefs and fears about untrustworthy people onto you. This sorting made me feel safe. However, I learned that the box I put people in was more a reflection of me, my fears, and Self-judgment, than the person I was judging and projecting my fears onto.

When we open our arms and care for the part of us that is afraid, hurting, full of shame, or feeling lost, guilty, or unacceptable, we become a safe place for ourselves. When we work with ourselves to embrace our disowned parts, we develop an inner understanding and compassion that extends to how we engage with others.

Behind every desire to profoundly accept ourselves, there is a story of Self-judgment or disconnection waiting to be seen and transformed. Life tends to isolate us from ourselves until we learn to see and let go of Self-judgment and profoundly accept the fears and beliefs that drive us.

We have all engaged in acts that are unacceptable to creating a healthy family, society, or relationship with ourselves. But a distinction between our unacceptable acts and the idea of ourselves as unacceptable is critical.

If the force greater than you always loves and accepts you, then you are always acceptable. You honor your undeniable worth when you profoundly accept your Self regardless of your mistakes and become responsible for your actions.

Say:
Even with my flaws, mistakes, bad choices, and fears, I ask to profoundly accept my Self and trust that I have innate value and worth.

How to Embrace Self-Acceptance

Self-acceptance is a synonym for freedom. My heart always seeks freedom, and when I am challenged, I assess the level of freedom I experience in my heart to know where I am. I know when dis-ease begins to mount. The first indication is a viselike tightness in my chest. The discomfort is sometimes excruciating. Here is what I've learned to do:

1. **Recognize the feeling** that indicates emotional concern is triggered. As soon as I recognize my pattern of overwhelm, I can begin to work with it directly. Overwhelm can be suddenly triggered for numerous reasons. I pay less attention to the why and bring my full presence to exactly what is happening inside me.

2. **Name it.** Breathing deeply helps me divert some of my attention to my breath, making the overwhelm less acute (though it may still be overwhelming). I begin to name all the dis-ease I am experiencing: the tightness in my chest; feelings of doubt, worry, and fear; and the level of intensity, if it is exceptional.

3. **Ground myself** by voicing my body's physical state, saying: *My feet are on the floor; my hands are on my lap; my back is resting against the chair.*

4. **Administer a compassionate touch and verbal acknowledgment** of my state: I massage the tightness in my heart area while making *even-though* statements: *Even though I am feeling this tightness in my chest, I profoundly accept myself and give myself permission to move beyond this state.* I do this for as long or as short a time as I need. I trust that every touch and *even-though* statement will help to soothe

me and send a message of Self-acceptance and courage to my subconscious and nervous system.

5. **Ask an EEQ** (effective and empowering question). EEQs open me to my future and a sense of possibility, and remind me that taking these steps is good for the human collective. I trust that the **EFFORT** (**E**xtracting **F**reedom **F**rom **O**ur **R**estricted **T**hinking) I invest in being conscious makes room inside of me and in the world for more freedom. I experience a rewarding sense of contributing to humanity when I take care of my Self in this way.

6. **Acknowledge any judgment** that tries to rise and get my attention during the process. I accept it, acknowledging it and accurately naming it, saying: *This is the habit of judgment trying to live through me.*

7. **Express gratitude** for the skill I have gained in being with myself in such profoundly accepting ways and for loving my Self enough to courageously be with my discomfort.

My Self-acceptance "treatment" is complete whenever I decide. I do not wait for all the feelings to settle. I go on with my life, and my emotions settle in the process of my living. Often, I become aware that the overwhelm has lifted.

We all have experienced our minds pulling us down the rabbit hole of worry, doubt, and fear. This is the nature of the brain's negative bias, but it puts us at odds with ourselves. Self-acceptance requires that we acknowledge and embrace the good and bad, comfortable and uncomfortable, aspects of ourselves and use them to grow if we choose. However, the surviving self sees discomfort as wrong and change as dangerous, and runs from, resists, and fights both. We must strengthen the thriving Self so we are prepared to manage the nature of the surviving self as needed.

When I acknowledge and accept how I am feeling or what I did, instead of running from myself, I always feel better—discovering more power inside me and feeling skilled at being my whole Self.

Learning to work with your surviving self with acceptance—without judgment or attack—is the goal. The path to this achievement is to remember that where you are is not who you are. If you find yourself the puppet of old patterns and beliefs, that is how it's been **up until now. From this point forward,** you can change this behavior without ever vilifying yourself or the behavior. **The way to such revolutionary change is the mindful act of accepting yourself, your feelings, and the situation.**

Self-Acceptance Is Self-Care

- Speak to your Self with profound acceptance and appreciation.
- Acknowledge your strengths, gifts, weaknesses, and flaws.
- Be willing to grow and change.
- Challenge your limiting fears and behavior.
- Listen to your Self and tell yourself the truth.
- Stop judging or comparing your Self to others.
- Express gratitude for your life.

There is healing power in this kind of intimate Self-care.

Belief Is NOT Necessary

When you begin this journey, you may not know how to profoundly accept your Self or believe in your value. Remember: The starting place for achieving profound Self-acceptance is to want it.

Wanting a better relationship with your Self guides your subconscious to realizations that support your intention. Practice Self-kindness with yourself: Every time you acknowledge your Self with respect, support, or appreciation, trust that your brain is taking notes and will strengthen the neural pathways that support creating consistent behavior. A part of your brain records your interest in your Self and, over time, will begin to interpret your kind thoughts about your Self or conscious contemplation of your struggles to know your Self and automatically generate good feelings about your Self. Allow your desires to live in your heart, and allow them to give you permission to be vulnerable enough to want a better relationship with your Self. Once the brain realizes you are engaging in new behavior regularly, it will work to find ways to turn your behavior into a more hardwired, automatic response. Although all conscious kind behavior moves you into an empowered relationship with your Self, all consistent unconscious Self-judgment and Self-attacks will disconnect you from your Self and turn your life into a breeding ground for isolation, low self-esteem, illness, and depression.

Say:
I intend to profoundly accept my Self and believe in my value.

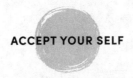

ACCEPT YOUR SELF

A Revolutionary Act
Be compassionate with the parts of yourself
you judge as flawed or unacceptable.

Inner Fitness Opportunity

Develop your skills for managing and rewiring internal overwhelm.

EEQs (Effective and Empowering Questions)

Ask aloud:

What must occur for me to become skilled at
managing my overwhelm with confidence?
How can I be more compassionate with my Self?

Forgive Yourself

———

I practice the art of forgiveness with myself and others.

THIS PRACTICE TURNS FORGIVENESS INTO A PROCESS OF Self-care and gives you the power to free your Self from any transgression.

You Have What You Need

Imagine yourself free of resentment, regret, or guilt; never again limited by what has happened in your life; and released from the pain and burden of hurtful events. This reality awaits, and the tools you need to claim this freedom cost no money. They live inside you.

Practice 3—*I embrace the idea that I am more than any challenge I face*—instills the idea that you can meet life's difficulties and, if necessary, pick yourself up, dust off any dirt, and stand tall. Practice 5—*I can choose a Self-empowering response in any situation*—reminds you that you get to choose whether you hold on to the pain of transgressions. This practice, Practice 9—*I practice the art of forgiveness with myself and others*—encourages you to choose forgiveness as a pathway to enhanced freedom and peace so that the hurtful behavior of others doesn't hijack your mind and emotionally imprison you.

A Not-So-Random Story About Acceptance

I lost my eldest sister in a fatal car crash before I was born. I asked my mother how she managed to get through the pain and whether she was angry at the driver. She said being angry wouldn't bring Carin back. Then she looked at me and said, "I had other babies I needed to care for." She added, "I was sad that the young man who hit Carin never apologized. I kept hoping he would."

As for how Mommy managed through the pain of losing Carin, Mommy said that in her mind she sent Carin away on a trip. Throughout the rest of my mother's life, she would periodically say out loud, "I wonder what Carin is doing." This was my mother's creative solution to a painful reality. This is how she used her mind to navigate her pain and her faith to believe there is more to life than what we see. She was not crazy. She was mindful. She knew her daughter wouldn't be returning. But my mother also knew she had two other children, my sister and brother, who needed her.

Mommy chose to be here for her babies—those who were here, and the ones yet to come. That was her purpose. Purpose helped her to accept the part of life that had cracked her heart, and to dare to love more and live fully, even with her loss. This was a powerful skill that Mommy would need later in life when she would bury two more of her children—Stevie and Marty.

Through her imagination, my mother found a rich life despite her loss. Carin was off on an amazing trip; Stevie was recovering from life's pain; Marty was taking a well-deserved rest. Mommy thought about her departed children often and would say out loud, *I wonder what they're doing?* Then she'd shake her head; look one of her living children, or grandchildren, or great-grandchildren in the eyes; and smile so wide it blessed everyone in our family. At ninety-one years of age, Mommy fiercely held hands across five generations. Until she died, Mommy thanked God regularly for having other children who needed her.

In my mother's approach to grief, I witnessed her extraordinary relationship with life. Often it was founded on forgiveness. Her forgiveness process had five steps:

1. **Acknowledge the hurt:** Mommy said she wanted to crawl into Carin's casket.

2. **Acknowledge how you wish things could be:** On top of her grief was the sadness that the young man never acknowledged her loss.

3. **Accept that life has bumped into you:** She knew anger would not help so she freed herself of it by choosing acceptance over blame.

4. **Make a Self-empowering choice:** Mommy shifted her focus from grief to a purpose and poured love into the babies who were still here and needed her.

5. **Have gratitude for what you have:** Every time Mommy smiled at her family, she was filled with gratitude.

We can't guarantee that life won't bump into us in painful or hurtful ways. But we can work to turn our lives over to a force greater than ourselves and discover that we are more than the drama and pain of life. This is what my mother did.

Say:
The worst day of my life never has to be the rest of my life.

But I Want to Be Angry

Forgiveness is not an easy choice when unforgivingness feels righteous and justified. If we have vowed never to forget what happened to us or the person or people responsible for our pain, then the anger, hate, or contempt we feel can provide a sense of purpose that leaves no room for forgiveness. Getting back at someone, living with coldness, and being emotionally unavailable can feel like winning. We feel powerful locking ourselves behind our hate and demanding the world to witness our pain. And, if we happen to hate our job, our marriage, or ourselves, revisiting hurtful events again and again acts as a great distraction. There's an odd dopamine high that can come with holding on to resentment and past transgressions.

As a young girl, I loved picking the scabs on my wounds until the wound bled again. Digging at the hard, crusty surface hypnotized me. I could pick, feel a little pain, and think simultaneously. Like picking at a scab, ruminating on people and events that have left us feeling wounded can be hypnotizing. Practice 9—*I practice the art of forgiveness with myself and others*—acknowledges forgiveness as a tricky endeavor that takes practice and imagination to disrupt the hypnotic nature of negative rumination.

Unforgivingness camouflages itself as regret, resentment, guilt, unkindness, bitterness, long-lasting anger, domination, and oppression. These emotions are rocks that weigh us down and take up inner space that dims our light and darkens our days because our creativity and imagination fall into the hands of the surviving self. Instead of thinking about what's possible and reaching for an empowered sense of Self, we ruminate on what's been taken from us, how unfair life is, and asking, without words, what we did to deserve such pain. Some of us think we are kicked so often that feeling like nothing and nobody becomes normal. Breaking our compulsion with negative rumination takes **EFFORT** (Extracting Freedom From Our Restricted Thinking) because it's the surviving self's nature to habitually revisit the painful, dangerous events that happen to us.

Say:
Achieving freedom in any area of my life takes effort.

A Bigger Truth Exists

Yes, life can challenge us with the most difficult parts of being human—betrayal, abuse, death. As painful and hard to swallow as it may be, the truth about the worst possible event still is this: *Life is bumping into life, creating more life.* How we respond is the only control we have. And it is best to respond intentionally because our response creates our future.

The hurtful moments, heinous acts, or other emotionally disturbing events that bump into us and don't kill us never have to be the end of our story. Reminding ourselves that *life is always bumping into life, creating more life* helps us remember to create distance between ourselves and the painful events that happen in our lives so that we can honor and respect ourselves and what we have been through without becoming identified with the pain. The simplicity of *life bumping into life* may not feel satisfying or easy to swallow, but it is a great starting point. Because it is the truth.

Say:
Life is simply bumping into life, creating more life.

We must cultivate an internal environment conducive to thriving—one that fosters resilience, growth, and freedom even in hellish circumstances. In a thriving environment, we will always experience a sense of openness. Openness provides the space we need for our untapped possibilities to move to the foreground of our hearts and minds. The power of our thriving and infinite qualities is always present in our lives, but it is easy to lose our connection to qualities like hope and possibility, and discard the idea of our being innately whole and undeniably worthy. We become distracted from the truth when drama and trauma take center stage.

For the qualities of our thriving Self and infinite SELF to move to the foreground and forgiveness to penetrate unforgivingness, two crucial things are necessary: (1) You cannot take even the hardest parts of life personally, and (2) remember that your truest Self is innately Creative, Resilient, Empowered to choose, Whole, and Worthy (**CREWW**).

When we start with the notion that we are innately whole and worthy, then in the harshest circumstances, no matter how excruciating, a part of us, no matter how small, can believe in that wholeness and worthiness. This perspective supports maintaining or developing confidence as you navigate any situation. Practice 9—*I practice the art of forgiveness with myself and others*—offers a powerful approach to creating the internal environment we need to heal and thrive.

The Truth About Forgiveness

Our lives are cosmic miracles. Our gifts are many. In addition to the gift of our CREWW, which generates infinite creativity and imagination, we are capable, intuitive, and full of possibility. We can, with our minds and hearts, transform every area of our lives. We are so much more than we have learned to appreciate. We each are a force to be reckoned with; the nature of the cosmos lights us from within and supports our very existence. Nearly every major religion and spiritual teaching states we are loved by a force that holds the universe.

Despite our unique fingerprint that proves we matter, we often treat ourselves like we don't matter and take the miracle of life for granted. We step over our Self, doubt and ignore our gifts, and live in fear instead of curiosity, doubt instead of wonder, and look for what's wrong instead of loving the joy of living. This is where forgiveness is needed. We must forgive ourselves for how easily we doubt our worth, judge ourselves, and devalue our gifts.

This attitude is the mistake we must forgive ourselves for: When a mate cheats; when someone we love dies; when we are treated violently, abused, or neglected; or when people treat us in mean-spirited and hurtful ways, we allow these events to define us, and we abandon ourselves. We let go of the CREWW version of ourselves and adopt feeling damaged, broken, not good enough, stupid, gullible, naïve, or insecure. Yes, something difficult or even tragic has happened, but on top of that pain, we add Self-attack, disrespect, abandonment, and rejection.

This is where Practice 9—*I practice the art of forgiveness with myself and others*—and Practice 8—*I ask to profoundly accept my Self and believe in my value*—can transform our lives. The way out of our misconceived relationship with ourselves and life is through forgiveness. We can take the radical step of forgiving ourselves for thinking of ourselves so negatively and treating ourselves and life with such reproach.

Creating forgiveness statements tailored to you, acknowledging how you have forgotten your innate wholeness and connection to your higher power, is called "forgiveness work."

Say:

I forgive myself for ever judging my Self as a victim.

I forgive myself for ever judging my Self as powerless.

I forgive myself for ever judging my Self as lost, broken, or alone.

I forgive myself for ever reducing my Self and life to a single moment.

I forgive myself for forgetting to dream despite my circumstances.

I forgive myself for ever giving up on my Self.

When you administer Self-forgiveness, notice that there is a profound difference between saying "I forgive myself *for being* [something]" and "I forgive myself *for ever judging myself as* [something]." When you forgive yourself *for being* something, you wrongly identify yourself with that thing or transgression. For instance, if you forgive yourself for being lazy, you are claiming "lazy" as your nature instead of seeing it as changeable behavior.

The capital-*S* Self is called out in forgiveness work to help us remember that the innately whole and worthy Self, which is an extension of our higher power, always deserves our reverence and care. Forgetting that the Self is more than any circumstance or moment is the mistake we forgive. Seeing ourselves as powerless when we are powered by the highest power is a mistake that can burden and ruin this precious gift called life. When we remember that the Self is more and that Self is our CREWW, there is no place within us for lesser surviving self identifications to live. Saying "I forgive myself for *judging my Self as . . .*" calls the mistake out clearly: We affirm the power and presence of the Self as our true identity and forgive our judgment and attack of the Self.

Ask:
What are the ways I have judged my Self?

The Choice
We can place our gifts in the hands of the surviving self and hold grudges and practice being unforgiving, or we can use our thoughts to heal, strive, and fulfill our purpose. But the latter requires us first to be curious and ask, *How do I apply creative skill and imagination to emotional hurt or trauma?* Answer: Define your Self as whole and unbreakable; allow the possibility of finding unexpected gifts, roadmaps, or healing within pain; and engage your difficulties like you are on a treasure hunt, allowing them to help you grow and expand.

Ask:
How can I be open to discovering unexpected healing inside my hurt, resentment, and unforgivingness?

Asking this kind of effective and empowering question (EEQ) in the throes of hurt may be the last thing you want to do. But asking is a powerful step. It signals willingness. Willingness is the opening needed for change to occur. It indicates that a part of you wants freedom more than revenge or feeling victimized. This opening, no matter how small, breaks through the wall of the surviving self and makes room for growth and a new way of seeing yourself and your circumstances.

Forgive Yourself First

The notion that you must "forgive yourself first" for the hurtful, hateful things others do is always a potentially volatile discussion in our workshop setting. I have seen people become fighting mad, walk out of a room, or cry uncontrollably because they interpreted "forgive yourself first" to mean *they* did something to provoke the bad behavior of another. Victims rightly and vehemently reject the idea that they are at fault.

It is easy to misinterpret "forgive yourself first" to mean "it's your own damn fault." So, hear me as I loudly and clearly proclaim: *Another person's bad behavior is not your fault, nor is it your responsibility.*

However, another person's unconscious behavior is not worthy of your time, hurt heart, or years of feeling less-than. Applying Self-directed forgiveness first helps you see the lie that another person has handed you and more importantly the lie about your capital-*S* Self that you have unconsciously taken hold of. Doing your Self-forgiveness for any lie that snags you as soon as possible is an efficient and Self-loving choice. This is the aim of Practice 9—*I practice the art of forgiveness with myself and others.*

Say:
Tending to my Self first means remembering the infinite SELF within and then rejecting any tendency to attack, doubt, or distrust that SELF.

Tend to Your Inner Child

Imagine your child coming home and telling you that the school bully had attacked them, and you tell your child that the bully's behavior now means your child is broken or less capable or viable. That response could be crushing and limit your wonderful child's sense of themselves and what is possible for them going forward. Where is your faith in your child? How does your child feel being so quickly discounted?

How would your child feel if you said something like this instead: Baby, you are innately creative, resilient, empowered to choose how you respond to that bully, and your higher power made you whole and worthy. That means you can't be broken. When mean people or bad circumstances bump into you and even knock you down, and you feel broken, you are never broken. You must remember that you carry within your DNA creativity, resilience, and the power to choose that the universe has placed inside you. Don't wait for someone to apologize and see the error of their ways. **Start talking to your Self. Forgive yourself.**

Having such a talk with your inner Self may not seem like the answer you need, but it establishes the important mindset that there is more to you and there is growth and life beyond any set of circumstances.

Ask:

How can I thrive beyond this experience?

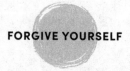

FORGIVE YOURSELF

A Revolutionary Act

Where there is the slightest bit of unforgivingness, forgive yourself for buying into the lie it has told you. Identify a purpose more powerful than the history of your unforgivingness.

Inner Fitness Opportunity

Discover the profound ability to accept where you are
and thrive despite the grief or pain you've withstood.

EEQs (Effective and Empowering Questions)

Ask aloud:

How can I forgive in the areas where I don't want to?

What must occur for forgiveness to penetrate
my heart and set me free?

Parent Yourself

———

I become a great parent and friend to myself.

T HIS PRACTICE TEACHES YOU TO PROACTIVELY TAKE CARE of your Self.

A Parent's Love

Imagine that you are headed home from a hellish day at work. You're feeling out of sorts, frustrated, and overwhelmed by life. You decide to stop by your parents' house. Your mom lights up as she sees you cross her threshold unexpectedly; she hugs you warmly, and you see and feel the joy your presence brings. Your father's joy is different; it shows up in how his body relaxes as he hugs you, knowing you are safe. You trail your mother as she moves around the kitchen. Being in your parents' presence just feels good. Your visit lasts for an hour or two. Hugging your dad goodbye, you feel love, trust, and a sense of security. You head home fortified and calmed by your parents' love. The earlier frustrations of your hellish day still exist but matter less. Feeling like you matter has made you stronger.

Now, imagine having this kind of loving relationship with your Self.

Only one thing is as important and meaningful as our relationship with our parents: our relationship with our Self. Practice 10—*I become a great parent and friend to myself*—reminds us that giving ourselves the love and care we need is as powerful as receiving it from others.

Whether you do or don't know firsthand the benefits of having great parents and friends in your life, from this point forward, let your idea of that love live in the background of your relationship with your Self and guide how you see, think about, and nurture your Self. With this simple strategy, you can heal and grow beyond old hurt, lovingly champion your Self, and *become a great parent and friend to yourself.*

Imagine the Life You Want

My mother lost her mom and dad when she was only six years old. She was reared by her grandmother until she passed, when Mommy was twelve. Then Mommy was treated poorly by her mean-spirited grandfather until an aunt stepped in, took mommy, and ushered her into womanhood.

For much of her young life, my mother mourned the absence of her parents' love. She turned to her imagination for comfort and poured countless hours into the daydream of being married and having a family. She imagined having four or five happy, healthy children and a house full of warmth and love that was also a meeting ground and safe place for neighborhood children. Anyone who didn't have a family was guaranteed a seat at her dining room table on holidays. Mommy's daydreams turned into the household I grew up in.

The Past Can't Stop You

Dreaming of an experience—filling our imagination with pictures and scenarios of how we wish things could be—is the only way to generate the experiences we want. Mommy's grandfather denied her ice cream when the truck came around, clothes when her old ones no longer fit, and the company of playmates. But he could not crawl into her head and stop the pictures and scenarios of a loving family that would become her life. Only *we* can stop ourselves from dreaming. Focusing our attention inward, thinking about what we needed, and reconciling what was missing from our parents' care is a personal and private act.

No area of life is off-limits or immune to the impact of a deliberate imagination: If we want better health, more purpose, joy, freedom, or peace, we need to start imagining it. When we dare to direct the force of our imagination and hope toward our hearts and imagine our hearts lighter and the empty places filled, we set in motion a better future that wants to make its way to us as much as we want it.

We must stop withholding and discounting the impact of giving ourselves our love and our ability to change our lives for the better. If you didn't get the love you needed from the parents you had, or in any other relationship, Practice 10—*I become a great parent and friend to myself*—is your call to action.

No one is left out because their parents weren't the best at parenting or because they had fair-weather or unreliable friends. Your inner Self is more powerful than your external circumstances; nurturing this Self heals, strengthens, and forges resilience, confidence, and Self-agency. You and your higher power become the force that moves your life forward.

Understandably, our hearts yearn for parents who care for our needs. But when they don't, we are not doomed. Within us is everything we need to live a better life. We can give ourselves the care we need. We can listen to ourselves, value and respect our Self, and even take twenty seconds a day to Self-soothe by wrapping our arms around ourselves for the benefit of our own touch. We mustn't blame ourselves or conclude we are unworthy because others can't or don't give us what we need.

Say:
I have not been left behind because of what my parents did or didn't do. It is impossible for me to be left out of my life.

The Expectation

We expect parents to prioritize their children because we believe that's what good parents do. But there are many reasons some parents behave less ideally or even violently: If a parent didn't experience being prioritized by their parents, or if they themselves were abused, they have no model for how they should behave. If a parent was reared as the center of their parents' universe, they might not have learned to see and value others. If a parent suffers with substance abuse or trauma and their Self-awareness is impaired, they may not be equipped to assess what is needed of them and to parent effectively. Each scenario is a case of life bumping into life. Ill-equipped parents bumped into you; however, they gave you the most important thing: life.

You can now effectively navigate from that starting point. You no longer have to take your parents' poor parenting, absence, or abuse personally. Strategies exist to help you move beyond the hurt. You can affirm your Self as **innately creative, resilient, empowered to choose, whole, and worthy, turn your life over to a force greater than you that loves you and responds to your heart, and ASK this force to help you to profoundly accept your Self and believe in your value.** You can use your Self-agency to become a great parent and friend to yourself.

At the Start

Being born into the world comes with only one guarantee: Life will bump into us, and something will be created. There is no certainty that what will be created will be best for us. This is why our ability to choose Self-empowering responses is critical. Activating Practice 10—*I become a great parent and friend to myself*—is choosing a Self-empowering response.

We slide into this world headfirst, knowing nothing about the people in whose arms we will land. Are they sane and happy? Will they be in our lives for the long haul? Will they love us as we need to be loved? Do they love themselves? Will we feel safe, know laughter, and feel prioritized, cherished, and encouraged to dream?

The parents we get will instill in us unconscious habits, familial patterns, and beliefs we have no say in. They will instigate ways of thinking that form who we are and what we remember and believe about ourselves. Many of us will be handed beliefs we must exchange for higher truths to become happy. But whatever we are handed, we must face an unavoidable reality: It is on each of us to create the changes we desire and the better lives we want. This is the support embedded in the 14 Practices and the specific promise of Practice 10—*I become a great parent and friend to myself.*

When something essential is left out of our care and we feel underloved or otherwise negatively impacted, the most efficient choice with the greatest chance of righting our misfortune is to become proactive: *Develop personal agency.*

Self-agency is realizing we have the power to change our lives and provide for our own needs. We exercise this power when we choose a Self-empowering response when life bumps into us. How we respond makes us producers of our story. If we tell ourselves things like "No one loves me," "I'm all alone," and "Enemies are around every corner," convinced that our narrative is true, we project our perspective onto the words and actions of others.

I worked with a woman who was convinced that the people in her life merely tolerated her. She longed for connection and a sense of belonging that never seemed to manifest. If someone disagreed with her, she was certain she was being attacked or put down. The more we talked, the more it was obvious to me that her way of seeing herself was at the root of her experience. She called herself names and judged herself as not being interesting or worth talking to and left herself out of conversations. She may have learned this behavior from her family, and if so, that was ignorant, uninformed parenting. She believed there was nothing she could do at this late date to change the way her childhood affected her life. But with the 14 Practices, she learned that her limited perspective could change. Today, she behaves toward herself using new parenting skills. She became aware of the narrative in her head and her actions toward herself, and she learned how to stop herself from perpetuating the bad behavior.

Say:

I can see when I am about to attack myself or perpetuate my old narrative, and I can choose not to speak the old words or engage the unsupportive behavior.

We all walk into rooms and encounter others, defaulting to our habits, hurting ourselves with the stories we tell ourselves. This stops when we exercise our ability to train ourselves to engage in new habits. The trick is to see how we project our story onto others and exercise our ability to change our story. We can give ourselves what we feel the world is withholding from us.

Say:

I can give my Self the time, attention, praise, appreciation,
respect, or care I want.
My love for myself is as powerful for my wellbeing as being
loved by another.

Beyond Family

A supportive family is comforting. But family cannot be the ultimate determinant of our resilience and sense of Self. Sometimes the
family we are born into is dysfunctional and unloving, and we all
eventually lose family members. Does this mean our lives are over
or forever unhappy? Everyone experiences loss of family, yet not
everyone is left devastated or destroyed. What allows some to rise
and thrive beyond the loss of family? We must dare to be curious
about how we can thrive beyond devastation. Curiosity opens us to
the idea that thriving beyond devastation *might be possible*.

Ask:

How can I thrive no matter my circumstances?

When we look deeper, a higher purpose and power is the in-
exhaustible resource that makes thriving possible despite our circumstances. When we adopt growth and expansion as the innate
purpose embedded in all life, this purpose allows us to skillfully
navigate when life bumps into us.

Our next step in processing difficulty or hurt is always the same:
Use the moment or circumstance to grow. When our commitment
to growth is primary, the problem is secondary. We approach the
problem ready to see how it can make our lives better. This mindset
allows us to address any problem with a sense of possibility in our

minds and hearts. This sense of possibility, no matter how faint, creates a crack in doubt or devastation through which the innately whole and worthy part of us can make its way to the surface.

When I lead with this growth mindset, I can hear my Self guiding my thoughts and actions like a parent or friend would, saying: *Honey, your job is to do your best. Remember that this situation or moment does not represent who you are. Your commitment to growth and healing and your courage are your wins. Your sense of worth does not come from getting this or anything; it comes from trusting in your purpose and growing in whatever way necessary to fulfill it.*

When we continually expand, we can love fiercely or experience deep hurt and use both to grow. There are many examples of people who have lost their entire family and found that their own resilience was more potent than their circumstances.

Say:
No matter the details of my circumstances, I can use them to grow and become more of my Self.

Adulthood

There comes a point in life when it doesn't matter what our parents did or did not do. The responsibility for managing the quality of our lives belongs to us. It would be nice if parents had parented better, but eventually, their mistakes cannot define us.

Five spiritual factors release our parents from blame:

1. Every human being is called from within to grow and expand. This is the nature of the universe and a cosmic edict. Every plant or life-form grows. To use the gift of life well we must expand our thinking and grow beyond where we are.

2. No matter how life has been up until now, every person can change for the better. Suffering can give way to relief, Self-forgiveness, and opportunity; it can point us in the direction of new choices and better ways of thinking.

3. Every human is equipped with what it takes to create a more fulfilling life—the ability to change our thoughts and behavior and rewire our responses. **EFFORT** (**E**xtracting **F**reedom **F**rom **O**ur **R**estricted **T**hinking) is our renewable resource that leads to change.

4. Life bumps into life, creating more life. We can be intentional about how we respond when life bumps into us. We can use the past intentionally to create our future.

5. Our higher power responds to our hearts (Practice 1). Asking for assistance in changing our lives (Practice 2) and embracing the idea that we are more than any challenge we face (Practice 3) are powerful first steps toward creating the change we seek.

Life does not come with an owner's manual. Parents wing it in many instances—holding their breath, doing what they were taught, and hoping for the best. This is true of the parents who come to the task wanting to do things right and those who are flying by the seat of their pants. It is impossible for anyone to know the intricate needs of another's soul when they barely know themselves or their needs.

We must take comfort in truisms: *Every parent did the best they could* and *If they had known better, they would have done better.* When we begin to extend this grace to ourselves and forgive ourselves for judging ourselves for things we did not or could not know, then we can extend this grace to our parents and their mistakes. Practice 10—*I become a great parent and friend to myself*—frees ourselves and our parents of the past and gives us permission to create a new experience by learning to deeply and profoundly love our Self.

A Partial Owner's Manual for Human Beings

If an owner's manual did come with life or parenting, here are seven parenting skills it would surely emphasize, along with how you can use these skills to become a great parent to yourself.

1. **Treat your child like they matter.** To be a good parent to yourself, treat your Self like your feelings, needs, and growth matter.

2. **How you speak to your child teaches them how to speak to themselves.** The words you use to speak to your Self matter. Putting your Self down for any reason is not good parenting. Become a good parent and friend to yourself, and choose a more Self-empowering way to speak to your Self.

3. **Your needs and difficulties are yours; work to resolve them so they do not become your child's responsibility or burden.** You are responsible for your growth. Acknowledge what happened that hurt you, what is missing that needs to be addressed or reconciled, and what is possible for your life. Blaming others for the difficulties they've handed you is unhelpful. Life bumped into you and gave you the parents and experiences you had. Your parents did the best they

could with the level of Self they had. You can choose a Self-empowering response and change your life for the better, from this point forward.

4. **Tell your child the truth so their resilience and intuition can be strong.** Telling yourself the truth allows you to practice operating from the truth. It fosters Self-trust and resilience. By developing an honest relationship with your Self, you learn to turn to it for your answers and to trust your intuition. You deserve to have this kind of confidence and trust with your Self.

5. **Instill the notion that your child is never alone and a force as big as the universe walks with them.** Contemplate the practice of turning your life over to a power greater than yourself. Strive to create a relationship with this power: Talk to it daily, ask for guidance and expect it to show up, and voice gratitude.

6. **If you use mistakes and challenges as navigational tools, your child will never know failure.** Acknowledge that you are a work in progress and aim to constantly evolve into the next best iteration of your Self.

7. **Constantly discover your Self.** You can't hold yourself responsible for what you do not know, but you are responsible for your growth and skills. You are full of the infinite possibilities of the infinite SELF. Use this lifetime to uncover more of your infinite nature. *Always see your Self becoming better.*

Falling Isn't a Problem

It is natural for parents to watch their children play and get hurt or try things and fail without concluding that their children are failing. Healthy parenting makes room for children to fulfill their potential and views children through a lens that is focused on the big picture—walking, talking, learning, and creating their best life.

Every parent accepts the reality that when learning to walk, children fall down. Those falls signal and celebrate the transition from crawling to walking to joyously running. When a child falls, parents would never automatically worry that their child will never walk or run. They know that falling isn't a problem.

You can nurture your Self, knowing that falling isn't a problem; it is the means by which you are moving toward your best life.

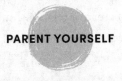

PARENT YOURSELF

A Revolutionary Act

Accept the most challenging, hurtful, or unacceptable
part of your life and use it to grow.

Inner Fitness Opportunity

With a growth mindset, you are always in the process of
fulfilling your innate purpose, on purpose and purposefully.

EEQ (Effective and Empowering Question)

Ask aloud:
How can I use this part of my life that I have judged
up until now to expand into my infinite power?

Make Friends with the Truth

—

I tell myself the truth about what happened,
my interpretation, how I feel, and what's possible.

THIS PRACTICE HELPS YOU ACCESS THE CLARITY AND power in telling yourself the truth.

Truth

Truth loves being seen, and seeing the truth feels good. It is a salve that vanquishes lies, helps calm the nervous system, and promotes healing. Truth is always in the background, waiting to enter and make our lives better, transforming emotional disturbance into understanding and personal power. We each are one realization away from greater clarity and inner freedom.

The challenge we face is confronting the unconscious or hidden lies, misconceptions, and judgments we carry that cause our self-doubt and unhappiness. Practice 11—*I tell myself the truth about what happened, my interpretation, how I feel, and what's possible*—is a four-part Self-inquiry that replaces internal disturbance with the salve of telling ourselves the truth, and from that **EFFORT** (Extracting Freedom From Our Restricted Thinking) gaining Self-understanding and greater personal freedom.

Truth 1: What Happened

Telling ourselves the truth begins with stating the facts about *what happened* that hurt us or got under our skin and separated us from our Self, thereby making us feel less confident or hopeful.

It is a mistake to think that *what happened* has to be a big traumatic event that makes separation an understandable result. *What happened* might be just a simple hurtful statement, or a series of little moments that undermine how we feel about ourselves. The size of the moment that pulls us away from ourselves does not matter. Any experience or event that leaves us feeling unworthy, worthless, not good enough, or estranged from ourselves must be acknowledged so that the repair that comes with telling ourselves the truth can occur.

If a "silly" moment keeps replaying in your mind, it is not silly. It is an event that you must acknowledge so you can make peace with it and reclaim your whole Self. Whether you perceive a moment as silly or traumatic, when you don't address its impact on you, that event can become featured in your mind and heart. If something hurts you or causes doubt, insecurity, or self-directed distrust, it is an act of Self-care to address such moments sooner rather than later. Even if it takes you years to acknowledge a hurt that you've been carrying, it is never too late to do so. (*Please note:* It is best to initially explore buried traumatic moments with a professional therapist.)

Practice 11—*I tell myself the truth about what happened, my interpretation, how I feel, and what's possible*—allows you to sit in your observer's chair and revisit the disturbing incident to see truths you might otherwise miss.

Say:
What happened in my life is important, but it is not the whole story of me.

Truth 2: My Interpretation

Telling ourselves the whole truth starts with accurately describing our experience. But the facts about what happened are never the whole story. They are the starting point, setting the stage and representing the circumstances. But seeing how we engage with the facts adds a layer of personal truth. Our interpretation of events plays a critical role in our experience.

In one of our workshops that takes a deep dive into Practice 11—*I tell myself the truth about what happened, my interpretation, how I feel, and what's possible*—a woman chose to explore an event concerning her father that happened when she was seven years old. Her mother had passed away, and her father had remarried quickly. She began to tell her story full of emotions and judgment. I stopped and coached her to stick with the facts. It took some time to sort through all the details of her story, but these are the basic facts she produced:

- My mother died.
- My father remarried.
- My stepmom had three children.
- I had to share my father's attention.
- I tried to share one of my drawings with him, and he said, "Not now, I have more than just you to consider."

Of course, the woman's experience included more details than these facts could acknowledge or reveal. So we revisited this list, leaving room for more of what was present but unconscious or unseen and needing to be revealed. I coached her to identify any *interpretation* of each bullet point that was part of her experience but not acknowledged.

Fact	Interpretation
My mother died.	God hates me.
My father remarried.	My father doesn't love me.
My stepmom had three children.	I am replaceable.
I had to share my father's attention.	I am not a priority.
I tried to share one of my drawings with him, and he said, "Not now, I have more than just you to consider."	I am an annoyance.

The workshop participant was surprised by her interpretations. For years she had felt like she didn't belong anywhere, but she didn't know why she felt that way. She was part of a blended family whose members seemed to get along well and care about one another. However, up until this exercise, the woman had judged herself as being petty because of the distance and quiet resentment she felt toward her stepsiblings, even though the siblings loved her genuinely. In the workshop, when her unconscious emotional experience of her dad remarrying was placed on the whiteboard, her internal experience—her *interpretations*—made sense, and she understood herself and her past reactions better.

Looking at just the facts of her experience would not have allowed her to see the other truths that shaped her experience.

When it comes to emotional experiences, we are often too overwhelmed, hurt, or triggered to remember the facts. We remember our reactions, which are fueled by our unconscious interpretation of events. Then, we assume that what we remember and feel are factual. But rarely are the facts or even our interpretation of the facts the whole truth. Facts are important, and our interpretations affect how we feel and respond. Only when these factors are clearly seen in tandem can the full truth be seen, and our emotional interpretations and stories challenged or updated.

Everyone has uncomfortable moments from the past that cause emotional distress. We experience pain when our interpretation of events is against ourselves. But remember, we are creators of our lives. When life bumps into us, we co-create our experience on the basis of how we respond. We have the power not to interpret events against ourselves and to change our habitual interpretations. Practice 5—*I can choose a Self-empowering response in any situation*—reminds us that we can change our interpretations by making new choices. Practice 11—*I tell myself the truth about what happened, my interpretation, how I feel, and what's possible*—teaches us to seek the whole truth.

Say:

I have the power to choose how I interpret events in my life.

Truth 3: How I Feel

How we feel matters. Feelings are our navigational system. They help us know where we are, where we want to go, whether we feel safe, and when we're hurt and need help. They protect us, move us forward, and remind us of when to take better care of ourselves. Feelings reveal information we can't get from just the facts, and they confirm or give greater insight into the impact of our interpretations. Yet we run from our feelings, ignore their warning signs, resent their intuition, and become angry with them when they reveal uncomfortable parts of ourselves.

I continued to work with the woman in our workshop to discover more about the impact the event with her father had had on her. I asked her to consider the facts and her interpretation together

and write down on the whiteboard the feelings—past or present—
that came up for her.

Her Past Feelings

Angry, enraged; feeling dismissed, forgotten, inconsequential;
hate for God, her mother, and her father; hopeless, small,
at risk, mean, feeling like a victim, bullied and backed into a
corner, profoundly sad, unhappy, lost, resentful, rejected

Her Present Feelings

Relieved, less burdened, sane instead of crazy, more open,
hopeful

There is a big difference between saying how we feel and being
caught in a fog of uncomfortable, negative feelings. The surviving
self prefers general fog over clearly naming feelings because general
fog doesn't require us to do anything. If we can't really see how we
feel, we can't address how we feel, and therefore we don't have to
take responsibility for where we are or seek to change. But once we
plainly state where we are, we can't pretend not to see or know that
we owe our inner Self more attention and care.

When we tell ourselves the truth about how we feel, without
Self-attack or blame, we treat our inner Self like a friend who we are
willing to show up for and listen to. Whenever our inner Self feels
like she or he matters, our confidence increases and strengthens.

Say:

Every time I take time to listen to my Self, I show my Self love.

Acknowledging how we feel is crucial to staying aligned with
ourselves.

Say:

The more I tell my Self the truth, the stronger my connection to my Self becomes.

We need never shy away from stating how we feel even if, on the surface, it seems negative. It is a misconception to think that acknowledging uncomfortable or negative feelings makes them more real. Keeping our feelings inside creates internal pressure, allowing the mind to ruminate and wander through our undefined malaise, making us vulnerable to negativity without calling it by name. Practice 11—*I tell myself the truth about what happened, my interpretation, how I feel, and what's possible*—will always open our hearts to something better.

Truth 4: What's Possible

Once you have a clear view of the whole truth, you are free enough to consider what's possible beyond the old events, interpretations, and feelings that have blocked your sense of possibility. Once you know where you are, the positive possibility is to move forward from there. What do you want? How might things change? What might you gain? When you ask yourself what is possible, you don't get stuck in the past because you are aware of your present situation. When you identify what's possible, you have a clear, compelling vision that can help move you forward.

Say:

No matter how tough things might be, a positive possibility is waiting to be realized.

Telling yourself your four-part truth is effective and efficient. Because no matter how uncomfortable the truth is, the whole truth isn't told until you acknowledge what is possible from this point forward. In the face of any difficulty, you can remind yourself that you haven't fully addressed the problem until you acknowledge a positive possibility within it.

Ask:
Now that I have greater access to the truth, what might be possible from here?

This mindset of considering what might be possible allows you to be open and to brainstorm possibilities without arguing with yourself about the most daring possibility that makes it to your list. Having the freedom to let your mind run wild and play just for the joy of fantasizing without feeling like you must commit to any particular direction opens you up. This play strengthens the thriving Self and makes regularly contemplating possibilities your new mindset. If the old way of seeing or navigating life revisits, looking to reclaim lost ground, the habits you will have established by engaging with Practice 11 will have made more room in your life for thriving rather than merely surviving.

*   *   *

In an infinite universe with a responsive higher power, beauty, growth, and greater freedom are waiting to emerge. Practice 11—*I tell myself the truth about what happened, my interpretation, how I feel, and what's possible*—creates space within the surviving self for new thoughts and considerations. Simply asking the effective and empowering question (EEQ) *How do I thrive more from this point forward?* makes space for something new to enter.

Ask:
What is possible for my life from this point forward?

It is easy to see possibilities when you follow this simple formula: Teach yourself to ask for and consider *the positive possibilities*, especially during challenging times. Every difficult or uncomfortable truth opens the mind to a positive possibility.

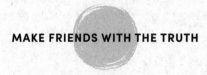

MAKE FRIENDS WITH THE TRUTH

A Revolutionary Act
Always seek the truth.

Inner Fitness Opportunity
The truth always creates a healing environment internally. Conscious and unconscious issues benefit from the calm and the clarity that truth generates. Truth aligns you with your Self.

EEQs (Effective and Empowering Questions)
Ask aloud:
How do I tell my Self the truth?
What is the deeper truth in this situation?
What must happen for the truth to be revealed?

Question Your Thoughts

———

*I realize I am more than my thoughts and feelings,
and not every thought or feeling needs to be indulged.*

THIS PRACTICE HELPS YOU CONSCIOUSLY ENGAGE WITH your thoughts and feelings rather than letting them dictate your life.

You Are the Boss

You are more powerful than the troublesome thoughts and feelings that compromise your internal state. Do not give ownership of your mind to the compelling but unsupportive noise in your head. It may be challenging, but you can choose how you engage with your thoughts and feelings. From this point forward, you can build confidence in your ability to work with your internal state more productively with Practice 12—*I realize I am more than my thoughts and feelings, and not every thought or feeling needs to be indulged.*

The more confident you become, the more you will test this concept and discover that your thoughts are not the boss of you. They are transient. With practice, the days of you being harassed and bullied by your internal state are numbered. You can learn to choose the thoughts and feelings you engage with, those you observe objectively, and when to step in and wrangle unruly thoughts and feelings.

You Choose

Every thought gains its life through you, and every thought can be starved of life by you. Thoughts are fleeting ideas. When we hold on to them, we give them life: A thought held tightly becomes a concept, then a belief, next a guiding principle, and finally a habitual way of being.

We hold on to thoughts tightly in areas where we suffer. Many people give up trying to change because their harassing thoughts have convinced them that the lies their mind tells are true. The mind is a powerful and busy thinking machine that never shuts down. But you can learn to put distance between yourself and the mind's incessant thinking.

Practice 12—*I realize I am more than my thoughts and feelings, and not every thought or feeling needs to be indulged*—helps reinforce the idea that you govern your internal state.

Say:

I am more than a mind.

I don't have to agree with or believe everything my mind says.

The Tireless Brain

We have all fallen asleep watching television and then awakened hours later to its nonstop broadcasting. Similarly, our conscious mind wakes up and falls asleep in front of the brain's nonstop thinking, remembering, and processing. When we are sleeping, our conscious mind goes "offline," but the subconscious never sleeps.

It is always processing our internal data. When we wake up, our conscious mind unavoidably reengages with our nonstop stream of consciousness.

Left to its own devices, the brain sees everything through the lens of survival. Meaning the surviving self is aptly labeled, and the negativity bias is real and formidable. The brain will naturally think, remember, and process our lives through the lens of the surviving self unless we consciously and actively step in and give our brains new data to process and learn from.

Say:

I am more than my negative mental tendencies.

You are powerful. Your interpretations of the good, bad, joyful, or hurtful events in your life have an impact. What you think, feel, and believe, and how you act and react, is data you give to your brain, which is constantly recording, assessing, interpreting, and processing everything in relation to you.

If we historically react a certain way, the brain interprets our consistency to mean this behavior is the correct response and will begin to repeat it on autopilot to free us up for the more important tasks of looking out for dangerous situations and keeping ourselves alive and safe. If we play a more conscious role and change our reactions, our brain will adapt accordingly.

I chatted with a man who was convinced he was a loser. His thoughts and feelings told him he was a loser. I did not see a loser. I experienced a man capable of being in a meaningful conversation. I knew that if he could contribute thoughtful insights in a conversation with me, he could be in a better, more empowering conversation with himself and stop indulging his habitual negative

Self-judgment. But he would have to decide to engage with himself differently and regularly.

When we consistently engage in a negative narrative of ourselves, we strengthen the mind's ability to quickly access and engage those thoughts. Our negative narrative habit is like any other addiction. We must hit a point where we want a new story enough to break the habit of following our old beliefs. Yes. This takes **EFFORT** (Extracting Freedom From Our Restricted Thinking).

Stepping over, running from, capitulating to, or gravitating toward our negative emotions generates feelings of powerlessness and sends our subconscious this message: *This issue is bigger than me. If I look at it, it will hurt and even destroy me.* That mindset places our thoughts in charge of our lives and reduces us to reactively responding to our thoughts and feelings. The only way to discover you are more than your thoughts and feelings is through confidence-building EFFORT. Providing tools and experiences that deliver this result is the aim of the Inner Fitness Project.

Say:
I can have Self-agency over my internal state.

You are powerful, and the EFFORT required of you is to deeply desire to see your Self as more powerful than your uncomfortable internal state.

Acknowledging this desire aloud to your Self helps condition your heart and mind to think new thoughts and say "NO" emphatically when old thoughts try to boss you around. This EFFORT helps you to strategically engage with your thriving Self and infinite SELF to feed the brain new thoughts, feelings, and data that support and install new behavior.

Assert Dominance

Thoughts are like dogs. Our furry friends come into our lives untrained, acting like they own us. And like all living things, dogs are driven by survival instincts. They love us for the food we give them but initially doubt our ability to keep them safe. It is our task to earn a dog's respect and trust. We gain our dogs' trust by giving them attention, creating boundaries, and disciplining them. We make space for new behaviors when we consistently interrupt our dog's bad behavior and affirm good behavior. Consistency helps the dog know what to expect and how to react; it eliminates uncertainty and creates the sense of safety a dog craves.

You must learn to train your errant dogged thoughts and feelings vigilantly. There's no magic pill. This is why the 14 Practices are called practices. Our relationship with ourselves takes the same level of EFFORT as forging a career, creating a successful marriage, rearing children, or working toward washboard abs.

Boundaries, Attention, and Discipline

Here's how you train your brain: boundaries, attention, and discipline:

- **Boundaries:** Dare to tell your brain what is acceptable to you rather than allowing it to control you. If you want your mind to be more of a friend and less terrifying, have a heart-to-heart with your brain and compassionately state what you need from it for a good relationship.
- **Attention:** The brain wants our attention. Its purpose is to take care of our safety. Let it know that you appreciate its intention. Pay attention when it works with you and not against you. Then, create a couple of key rules. For example: Speak kindly to me, and I will listen. If you try to intimidate,

bully, or run over me, I will ignore you altogether and only pay attention to the thriving Self.

- **Discipline:** Police what you let come into your mind and out of your mouth. Stop talking about your core issues in the same old way. When the mind is egging you on, entreating you to say something negative or Self-defeating, withdraw your energy from the mind and hold your tongue.

Every person is different. You will have to try different approaches to determine how to work with your mind more effectively. The amount of effort required varies from person to person and brain to brain. However, all EFFORT, whether successful or not, sends your brain the message that you intend a better, more empowered relationship with your Self. Each EFFORT sends your brain new information. The more consistent and repetitive your behavior, the more you will build and strengthen a new neural pathway.

Incremental increases in our ability to wrangle and manage our internal state embolden us to challenge more oppressive thoughts and feelings.

Say:

I ask to realize I am more than my worst thoughts and most challenging feelings, and ask for support in consistently engaging in new behavior.

My Experience

Sitting in my observer's chair, I became conscious of a tug-of-war that ensued often between my intuition and my compulsion to indulge my thoughts and feelings by telling a "story" in a way that fed my brain negative energy, reinforcing my thoughts and feelings. The telling of the story ignited all of the troubling feelings tied to my history of struggles and disbelief, especially when I was using the story to validate my perspective or gain confirmation from others that my conclusions and feelings were justified.

However, my intuition warned me not to tell these stories. It told me to resist talking about that certain problem or person. Intuition whispered to me: *Refusing to engage starves the story of the energy it needs to stay alive.* Often, I ignored that intuitive whisper and launched into the story or problem in the same old ways. Each time, I found my Self filled with the same old negative, blaming energy. I was right back where I didn't want to be, and the story was smiling, proud that it had strategically survived to be told again. Finally, after repetitive EFFORT, intuition won. I didn't indulge in the story, and I felt empowered. Since that day twenty years ago, whenever a story is egging me to *Just tell it*, *Say it*, or *Do it*, I choose instead to keep quiet and remember that **not all thoughts or feelings need to be indulged**.

A Not-So-Random Story About Negative Thoughts

Before being introduced to inner fitness and Tina, my thoughts left me feeling like I was doomed to be unhappy. I had more negative than positive thoughts. I told myself that something was wrong with me because I would have such a difficult time stopping my negative thoughts. My harsh Self-judgment made me depressed and angry.

When I was at my lowest, having just experienced deep pain around a breakup, the loss of which triggered all my losses in the past, I felt overwhelmed and had thoughts about killing myself.

A friend suggested I speak with Tina, and she helped me understand that I truly am more than my thoughts or feelings. I learned to step outside myself and look at what was going on inside of me under the layers of thoughts and feelings. I learned to be gentle with myself and embrace my humanness. I started allowing my thoughts and feelings to pass through me instead of judging them. I learned to float above myself and say, "Well, isn't that interesting? I'm thinking those thoughts or feeling a certain way." That helped me get distance and allowed me to separate myself from my emotions.

I learned I could accept that I was having a negative thought or feeling, acknowledge it, and send it on its way. My thoughts and feelings did not have to stick to me like superglue.

Now, regularly, I remind myself that I am not my thoughts or feelings, and my life is so much better because of it.

You Are in Control

You may not choose every thought you think. But you choose the general direction and tone of your thinking. The chooser is always more powerful than the thing being chosen, because you can say "yes" or "no" or accept or reject the thing as you choose. Practice 12—*I realize I am more than my thoughts and feelings, and not every thought or feeling needs to be indulged*—guides your thinking and helps keep you mentally and emotionally strong.

Say:

The more I challenge the habit of being me, the more I uncover the beauty and power of my authentic Self.

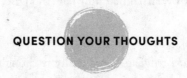

QUESTION YOUR THOUGHTS

A Revolutionary Act
The revolutionary act is to hang in there through internal
discomfort to achieve the change you desire. Every effort to
be with your troubling thoughts and feelings moves you closer
to the day you wake up and think and feel differently.

Inner Fitness Opportunity
Discover that the thriving and infinite range of
Self is a reliable and powerful resource.

EEQ (Effective and Empowering Question)
Ask aloud:
What does it mean that I am more than my thoughts and feelings?

Honor Your Process

———

I recognize that growth and healing are processes, and I compassionately allow myself and others the time we need.

THIS PRACTICE TEACHES PATIENCE, SELF-COMPASSION, and trust.

Wellbeing Follows a Process

It takes time to grow into the person you want to become and to heal the parts of you that need your attention and compassion. Unlearning or overriding ingrained habits takes time. This is work that cannot be rushed. However long the journey takes, the ultimate win is the discovery of the hidden power within your Self. Practice 13—*I recognize that growth and healing are processes, and I compassionately give myself and others the time we need*—reminds you that **you are worth the journey**. Healing is possible, regardless of the nature or age of your wounds or challenges. You can become better and stronger in every area of your life. You can do this because healing anything in your life begins with your relationship with your Self. And you can learn to take charge of that. You can seek guidance, ask for help, show yourself compassion, and give yourself grace. Everything else you need to become the person you want to be will be figured out through your growth and healing process.

Trust the Process

Trust the process were words I hated hearing at the start of my journey to my whole Self. Often, I wanted to shout *HOW*? *How* do I trust the process when I don't know what the frickin' process is? *How* do I change when I don't know *how* to change, and I doubt change is possible?

I couldn't see beyond my frustration, fear, and anger. Then, one day, I had three back-to-back aha moments:

1. If I can rely on Practice 1—I *practice turning my life over to a power greater than me that loves me and responds to my heart*—then acknowledging my desire to change is the most important action I can take. Filling my heart with desire gives the universe something to respond to.

2. Of course, I will doubt the process along the way. Fear, frustration, and anger anchor the surviving self, constricting our ability to see beyond a problem or limitation. Doubt doesn't have to stop me. I can understand that it is the nature of the surviving self to doubt. Instead of beating myself up, I can expect doubt to rear up and be ready for it.

3. Yet, even when I am distracted by the surviving self, the thriving Self and infinite SELF are present and active. I realized that even in my frustration and overwhelm, my thriving Self is present enough for me to ask an effective and

empowering question (EEQ): *How do I trust the process?* Yes, I was angry and frustrated and even internally shouting, but I also was asking an effective and empowering question, and the higher power always listens.

These thoughts brought a smile to my face. I was doing the work, even while fighting with my Self and life. I was growing and healing despite appearances. A part of me was present and hanging in there despite wanting to give up. I was "anchoring" new behavior.

Trust the process is easier said than done because, by the time we hear this guidance, a part of us is already in the grips of the surviving self and disconnected from our calm and rational problem-solving thriving Self mind.

Practice Trusting Your Self

Trusting the process begins with trusting our Selves **within** the process. You don't have to have an answer for your discomfort or know which direction to take. Just trust your Self when it wants to feel or do better. Then force yourself to ask how feeling better is possible, and your thriving Self's curiosity will open you to answers.

Ask:

How can I trust my Self?

How can I be kind to my Self, show my Self compassion, dream, and keep getting up despite my doubts?

We must remember that judging our Self puts us at risk of disconnecting *from* our Self and falling into a darker, more disconnected-from-Self place.

Revisit the 7 Laws of Self and allow these laws to guide how you see and engage with your Self:

Law 1: You have innate purpose and worth.
The goal: Stop trying to be "somebody" and instead be your wonderful, unique Self.

Law 2: The Self comprises your thoughts, feelings, and beliefs and creates your life's stories.
The goal: Adjust your thinking to interact with your Self more consciously and create your life more intentionally.

Law 3: A strong inner Self strengthens every area of your life.
The goal: Practice internal behavior that strengthens your relationship with your Self.

Law 4: You are connected to your higher power through the Self and can continually improve your life.
The goal: Learn to trust that you are connected to your higher power from within you.

Law 5: The Self must be nurtured to thrive.
The goal: Nurture your Self so that you can grow beyond your limiting beliefs and narratives.

Law 6: Unnurtured, the inner Self defaults to ingrained reactionary survival instincts.
The goal: Learn to see and interrupt your reactionary behavior.

Law 7: The inner Self is more powerful than external circumstances.
The goal: Discover the unseen and unengaged power within you.

When you ask how, you are spending time healing your Self.

Here's a supportive way to think about trusting the process going forward using TRUST as an acronym:

T: Treat your Self well.
R: Remember to turn to the thriving Self.
U: Understand the negative doubting nature of your surviving self.
S: See and stretch beyond where you are to whatever degree you can.
T: Think about positive possibilities.

Say:
Trusting the process begins with trusting my Self.

Ask:
How can I remember to embrace my worth and trust my ability to grow and heal?

Accept the Process

The journey to growth and healing is not a straight line. Yet, I yearned for and quietly demanded an easy path. I took the stance that life **should** follow a straight line that feels safe and guarantees the comfort I (my surviving self) wanted. But the comfort of the surviving self rarely allows life to progress. Living this way just eases our terror of the unknown by allowing us to maintain our less fulfilling but comfortable known habits and to repeat history.

My revolutionary act was to see that every time my surviving self threw a tantrum, wanting life to be easier, I was telling my Self that I couldn't handle life as it was, feeling like a victim, and needing something outside my Self to save me or make things better.

But the thriving Self that focuses on what's possible and the infinite SELF that affirms me as innately purposeful were patiently waiting for me to turn in their direction and engage. With practice, turning to this higher range within me became my default response.

We can be so focused on wanting to feel good and avoid discomfort that we miss the internal strengthening and resilience that discomfort teaches.

Discomfort is part of the process that moves life forward. It deserves our understanding, patience, and tolerance. In avoiding purposeful discomfort, we trade growth and internal expansion for what is known and feels safe.

The revolutionary act is to accept that the "no pain, no gain" mindset of physical fitness applies to building inner fitness and finding joy in building internal grit.

Say:
Pain in the name of gain leads me to the next better version of my Self.

Sit with Discomfort

Sitting **with** discomfort is different from sitting **in** discomfort. Sitting **in** discomfort can feel like Self-assault—full of Self-judgment about who you are and what you did or didn't do.

Sitting **with** discomfort is a purposeful act. Discomfort indicates the need to resolve something internally. Discomfort visits us for a reason—Self-care is needed. The openness and trust of your thriving Self courageously invites discomfort in and allows it to have its say. No running, avoiding, or feeling wrong. Listen to this part of your Self like you would a friend. Then work with your thriving Self and give it time to grow and heal.

The surviving self avoids looking within because habitual Self-judgment makes it afraid of what it might discover. The thriving Self sits with discomfort, curious and dedicated to growth and healing. The infinite SELF holds the memory of your whole Self and is the reminder that you are more than your history. Pain and discomfort are not who you are. They are where you are.

Say:
Compassionately working with discomfort turns it into a moment in time instead of a forever state. Discomfort is not who I am. It is where I am.

Pay Attention to Your Self

The growth and healing process is more than tending to the wounded parts of us. It extends to healing our unconscious disconnection from our inner Self. What did your authentic Self want to do that it was robbed of doing? How were the desires of your Self stifled?

Your answer may not be a big, obvious relinquished dream like a romantic relationship or career. It can be a simple missed opportunity—like wanting to stomp barefoot in the rain but something or someone stopping you, wanting to sing in the school talent show but shyness not allowing it, or neglecting to say I love you to a dying loved one. Lost moments matter if they teach you to hold back and not explore your potential.

You can tell the difference between the moments that mattered and the ones that did not. The ones that mattered left you with the feeling of having cheated or abandoned your Self in some way. You can revisit those moments that you remember and heal their loss by acknowledging them and forgiving yourself for giving up on your Self. You can do this with any memories or feelings that come up for you from any area of your life.

Say:

I forgive myself for letting go of important parts of my Self and
I vow to make room for my whole Self going forward.

Patience

A simplified understanding of how change happens can help you
exercise patience with your growth and healing process.

The brain can adapt and change throughout our lifetime. This
means you can change old habits and create new ones in any area of
your life. New habits are a function of repetitive behavior. It takes
about ten thousand repetitions to create a new neural pathway to
change an old habit. Therefore, you must practice a new behavior
ten thousand times or more to reprogram the old pathway and create a new behavior.

Every time you sit with your discomfort and respond to it differently, you create a new neural pathway that supports a different
way of thinking. And one day, your new habit will kick in and
become your new default as long as you continue to practice the
way of thinking and responding that caused and will maintain the
change.

You must practice patience until you have given the change you
want enough time to become established. So, breathe and stop com-
plaining about the past or resenting how things are. That behavior
will only strengthen habits you no longer want. Instead, begin to
think about and respond to life with the belief that your old responses can change. Be vigilant because the old habit can reengage
if you reawaken it by reverting to old behavior. Just like the saying
goes, we never forget how to ride a bike; what we learn lives on
in us. Our power lies in which Self we allow to engage. Growth
and healing are processes that require you to engage with your Self
thoughtfully, compassionately, and consistently. Practice 13—*I rec-*

ognize that growth and healing are processes, and I compassionately give myself and others the time we need—gives yourself time to heal.

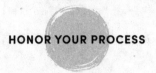

HONOR YOUR PROCESS

A Revolutionary Act
Every time you are about to judge your Self or someone else for a habit, say, "Growth and healing are processes, and I compassionately give myself and others the time we need."

Inner Fitness Opportunity
Develop compassion for yourself and others.

EEQs (Effective and Empowering Questions)
Ask aloud:
How can I let go of my frustrations and judgments regarding my growth and healing processes?
What must I see or where might I look to receive more insight into my growth and healing?

Find Your Community

———

I cultivate social connections where I feel safe, seen, and heard.

THIS PRACTICE ENCOURAGES YOU TO LOOK FOR A COMMU-
nity that supports your growth and cares about your happiness.

Discover Your Self with Others

You are designed to thrive; like a seed placed in the ground or womb, you are meant to grow into the life that awaits within you. From your birth to death, infinite potential lives inside you. Your historical challenges and past habits do not diminish your potential; they distract you from it. Therefore, keeping your eye on what's possible for your life is the surest way to find fulfillment. Keep in mind, you can never fulfill **all** of your potential because your potential is infinite. This life and your body are finite. With good tools, you can strengthen your thriving Self, awaken dormant potential, and experience more of what's possible for your life. Practice 14—*I cultivate social connections where I feel safe, seen, and heard*—shows how to identify people and create environments that support you in reclaiming or becoming your freest, most empowered Self.

A Safe Community

Everyone needs a safe place where they can hear their voice, speak their heart, and reclaim their whole Self. Obtaining information that helps you better understand your Self and engaging with practices and social environments conducive to thriving is the path to your internal freedom and potential.

Community is defined as a feeling of fellowship with others who share common interests, attitudes, and goals.

Inner fitness requires more from a community than like-mindedness. Your goal is a "safe community" where interactions honor you. When this mindset leads, each interaction is filled with respect, active listening, understanding, authenticity, and acknowledgment of another's innate worth and beauty, regardless of your differences, points of view, or emotional challenges.

A safe community is a place where others show up for your Self in the spirit of community. You can speak openly about your life and needs without fear of judgment, receiving unsolicited advice, or having others project their experience or beliefs onto you. The **community meets you where you are**, allowing you the time and space you need to reclaim your Self from life's misconceptions and lies. This time with your Self strengthens your **thriving Self** so you grow into more of your potential.

Most importantly, a safe community looks forward; it does not lead with who you were, what you've done, or what's happened in your life. Instead, it affirms your innate value and what's possible for your life from this point forward, and encourages and applauds your growth.

Say:
A safe community allows me to access more of my Self.

Being Seen and Heard

Research shows that feeling seen, listened to, and heard is funda-mental to wellbeing and impacts overall happiness. These feelings make us feel capable, which allows for an enhanced sense of per-sonal possibility and usefulness, and is the foundation of our ability to thrive. These benefits underscore the importance of employing Practice 14—*I cultivate social connections where I feel safe, seen, and heard.*

The work of psychiatrist Irvin D. Yalom helps explain the benefi-cial impact of feeling safe, seen, and heard. He discusses the concept of universality, which refers to the realization that our life experiences, though unique to us, are common human experiences. Listening to another's story and seeing ourselves in their experience validates our own experience. Through another person's story, we feel known be-cause "someone else knows my experience." This recognition reduces the stress of feeling different, alone, and disconnected from others. There is comfort in knowing that others struggle with the same chal-lenges we face. Seeing ourselves in another's story allows us to legit-imately trade feeling alone for a sense of validation and belonging.

Science Says

Numerous studies have confirmed that feeling seen, listened to, and heard leads to increased life satisfaction and overall well-being, greater levels of empathy and emotional intimacy, higher self-esteem, and lower stress, and supports building positive re-lationships.

The Inner Fitness Project defines a safe community as including trusting that each person has within them the answers they need to feel, do, and be better. The community's role is to be a place where its members can find their answers by sharing their story, looking within, and listening to themselves.

Say:
The answers I need are inside me, and I can discover them by spending time with my Self.

A Journey of Self-Trust

The power of community and the need for social connections where I felt safe, seen, and heard had to sneak up on me for me to see how much I needed the breakthroughs they provided.

I come from a close family where I grew up feeling safe, seen, and heard. I trusted my family to be there and root for me. However, Practice 14—*I cultivate social connections where I feel safe, seen, and heard*—taught me to trust the internal freedom and benefits gained from a safe and trusted community and made me more whole.

I used to keep many areas of my life unnecessarily private. Things that didn't need to be secrets were kept close to the vest out of habit. Today, as a trusted confidante to many, my ability to never divulge the stories entrusted to me serves me. But the closed-mouthedness I practiced into my forties was unnecessary secrecy that left me somewhat removed from others and from my Self. I liked people. But from listening to older folks, I learned to not want people "all up in my business." I chuckle while writing this because, after listening to so many people's stories over the years, I realize I never had much "business" to speak of. In other words, my learned behavior created an unnecessary distance between others and myself. My best explanation for this is that the surviving self, unmanaged, creates distance between us and the world because that is the safest and most manageable scenario for survival. We keep our tribe close and keep an eye on everyone else. But being in inner fitness workshops gave me permission to expand my notions of safety. The more I trusted my Self and led with *I embrace the idea that I am more than any challenge I face* (Practice 3) and *I can choose a Self-empowering response in any situation* (Practice 5), the more I could look to my Self for safety and trust in my ability to navigate my circumstances. The more I understood about the human condition and how the brain and nervous system operate, the less personally I took life and the less concerned I was with people knowing "my business." I was discovering that the human experience was the same for everyone. The specifics varied, but the challenges of knowing one's Self, managing the surviving self, healing, and being emotionally present, honest, and authentic were everyone's challenges.

Being in workshops, listening to others' stories, and experiencing Dr. Yalom's universality concept firsthand, I saw how shame and secrecy stunt our ability to thrive. Hundreds of people held secrets and stories related to events that often were out of their control. When we indulge in narratives that frame us as unacceptable, we violate the precept of our innate worthiness, making our fear of life greater and the surviving self stronger. This curtails the growth and expansion of the thriving Self.

Growth and thriving are tied together. No matter where we start, growth is needed and necessary to thrive. Whether they start with a great family, are alone and orphaned, or feel challenged or blessed, each person will need to grow from wherever they start to connect more deeply to their innate worth and personal possibilities.

Say:
Embracing my innate worth and potential is a lifelong process of growing and expanding.

Compassionately connecting with others taught me to be more compassionate with my Self. My thriving Self wanted and needed more time. I began to climb into the observer's chair and curiously look for my limiting **beliefs, patterns, and judgments** (Practice 4), courageously interrupting unhelpful patterns to make my potential more accessible.

There is honor and courage in using this lifetime to grow through tough times and shake free of old lies and baggage. The quickest way to achieve growth is to have safe, positive communities that support Self-growth.

Therapy, Friends, and Family

A "safe community" takes many forms. All are valuable when they align with the core premise behind the 7 Laws of Self: Your inner Self matters and you have innate purpose and worth.

A Thought

Strengthening your inner Self, letting go of the lies that stunt growth, and reclaiming your innate right to feel, do, and be better is the fastest path to your whole Self.

Having a good therapist can be an empowering way to experience a safe community: The therapist's office is welcoming, and the environment is free of judgment. My experience with therapy allowed me to see the unconscious hurts that manipulated my thoughts and feelings. Two years of therapy cleared the landscape for me to adopt a Self-reflective lifestyle of looking within for answers.

Inner fitness practices—understanding the **Three Selves**, discovering my learned behaviors, setting a standard for my relationship with my Self using the **7 Laws of Self**, and mindfully engaging with the **14 Practices**, as well as other prompts in this book—allow me to proactively maintain a healthy relationship with my Self.

Friends also helped me reclaim my **Self**. My girlfriend group of seven spiritually focused women became my first safe community outside my family. We all were committed to feeling, doing, and being better in our lives. Turning that commitment into a support group made sense. We referred to our group as the **Circle**. We agreed that we could benefit from feeling safe, seen, and heard by people we trust.

Whether it's a friend or confidant who lends a listening ear, a therapist, a support circle, a random person on the street, or simply reading a book like this one, conversations from the heart give you space to reclaim your Self and grow into your potential. As you grow into more of your Self and adopt new habits of Self-acceptance, you decide what you need and what parts of your life you want to share and with whom.

You can assess if a person or environment qualifies as a safe community using these simple metrics:

- You **FEEL** accepted.
- You **FEEL** like the person has your best interest at heart.
- You **FEEL** respected and never judged.
- You **FEEL** loved or appreciated, and care is never withheld.
- You **FEEL** empowered to be your Self.
- You **FEEL** acknowledged for your gifts and never resented or negatively compared to others.
- You **FEEL** interactions are authentic—free of gaslighting and lies.

- You **FEEL** trust for community and disagreements never violate the trust between you.

Say:
I can determine if I am in a safe community by assessing if I feel accepted without judgment, especially during disagreements.

Building a safe relationship with your Self turns your gut into a reliable resource. When we like, love, and respect our Selves, value our growth, and believe in our innate purposefulness and worth, we understand the importance of honoring our Selves. Trust your gut. You can sense and feel if a person or environment is supportive and worthy of you or not. People who don't honor you don't have to belong in your life. You get to choose. Either way, you can keep growing into more of your infinite potential.

Say:
Building a safe relationship with others begins by learning to be a safe place for my Self.

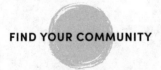

FIND YOUR COMMUNITY

A Revolutionary Act
Choose a safe place (therapist, support group, or friend) to share something you have not yet shared with anyone else. Set a time goal in which to do this.

Inner Fitness Opportunity

Speaking aloud about this in a safe place will feel like
a weight has been lifted. Hopefully, the experience
will become addictive until there is nothing, or very
little, that you carry with shame or judgment.

EEQs (Effective and Empowering Questions)

Ask aloud:

How can I find a safe place where I can experience my possibilities?

What must I realize to become my whole Self?

From This Point Forward

———

THE INNER FITNESS REVOLUTION IS REAL. BY ENGAGING IN actions that teach you to thrive, you can free yourself of baggage, uncover your wholeness, and experience more freedom and joy.

I know inner work is hard, but it is also exciting, liberating, and a different type of fun.

The stories that follow in "The Practice" exemplify this.

The tools I've shared with you make inner freedom accessible. They lead with the premise that you have innate purposefulness and worth. The Inner Fitness Project approach to personal wellbeing helps you recognize your innate ability to thrive and improve your life gracefully.

The 7 Laws of Self, Three Selves framework, and 14 Practices support thriving. By cultivating an internal environment conducive to thriving, you can change your life and free yourself in rewarding ways.

Your call to action is to imagine feeling fully alive, excited, and capable of navigating life, even in challenging times.

Kudos for taking the time to read this book
and show up for yourself.
You matter.

THE
PRACTICE

Real stories of growth and freedom.

Aida: A Difficult Mother

I GREW UP WATCHING OPRAH. I HAVE ALWAYS YEARNED FOR more. I loved self-help books, and I frequently read them to be a better version of myself, the version God created me to be. When COVID-19 hit in 2020, a sister-friend recommended the audiobook for *The Little Book of Big Lies*. I listened to it four times. I felt the book was written for me, and I ordered the hardcover and completed the inner fitness practice exercises at the end of the chapters. On the audiobook there was an invitation from Tina saying to come and hang out with her on Instagram or TheInnerFitness Project.com. I logged on and found all the workshops that were offered, including Wellness Wednesday. I joined my first Wellness Wednesday Zoom meeting on October 8, 2020, and I have been attending since then.

I was born in 1973 in the Ethiopian countryside to two teenage parents. I was told I was conceived in the back of a car at a high school party. My mother was seventeen years old, the oldest of all her siblings. She was very studious. When she found out she was pregnant, she was devastated and, I am sure, scared. As she explained the story to me, she told me that she wanted to have an abortion. However, she was told she was four months pregnant, and it was too late. She hid her pregnancy from everyone, including her mother. Her parents were divorced at the time, and she attended a boarding school. She told her dad that she was stressed from school and she needed a break. She went to see her grandmother who lived on a farm. She delivered me in the barn. When her grandmother heard a baby crying, she thought that one of the maids had a baby. She came running only to find out she was a great-grandmother.

My mother told me that she wanted to give me up for adoption, but her grandmother refused. Looking back, I think my mother always viewed me as her biggest mistake. It was easier to get rid of me and pretend I never existed than to disappoint her family.

She left Ethiopia when I was three weeks old and moved to New York with her uncle to attend school. When I was six years old, she found my dad, who was living in California then, and informed him he had a child. He called his parents in Ethiopia and told them to contact me. I look exactly like my dad, and when his mother saw me, she cried and asked if she could raise me. I lived with my father's family until I left my country. I am thankful for my paternal grandmother. For the first time, I felt somebody wanted me. It was wonderful being surrounded by four grandparents and a great-grandmother. Even in the absence of my parents, they filled the void with their unconditional love.

All that changed when I was ten. I moved to Washington, DC, to live with my mother. Even though she had me at a young age, she obtained her master's degree in economics from Syracuse University and secured a remarkable job at a prestigious financial institution. I was looking forward to finally living with my mother.

She was able to take care of me financially. But living with my mother was not what I had imagined. I was taken from an environment where I was loved and cherished to one where I would be physically, verbally, and emotionally abused.

I missed my Ethiopian family immensely. I decided to call them to hear my grandmother's voice. When the phone bill arrived, my mother asked me if I called them. I told her no because I feared what she would do. My worst fear came true. She hit me at least twenty times with the metal end of a belt. My back was covered with blood and bruises. She told me to stand up against the wall all night while she slept. I must have fallen asleep standing and ended up falling on the floor in the middle of the night. She stepped over me to use the washroom as if nothing had happened. I always asked myself, *What kind of a mother does that?* This happened thirty-seven years ago, and I remember it like it was yesterday. I yearned to return home to be with my grandparents, away from the nightmare I was living. To make it worse, everyone who knew what was going on looked the other way.

My mother belittled me in every way she could and told me many lies. One of her favorite lines was "The day you were born was the worst day of my life." I often asked God if my mother and father did not want me, why I was born. But through it all, I am so grateful to my grandmother for taking me to church from a young age. In times of trouble, I grabbed my Bible and found comfort in God's words or just held it close to my heart. I believe God brought me into this world for a reason. I promised myself that if I became a mother, I would tell my children every day how much I love them. How grateful I am for them. I am going to be a better mother. I will give them everything I never had. I will provide them with a home that is full of love, peace, laughter, and security. God has blessed my husband and I with two amazing children. I was able to become the mother that I always wished I had. My children benefited. They both know how much they are loved and that they are lovable.

* * *

My biggest realization on my inner fitness journey was when Tina explained: "The mean and damaging things others have told you are lies. Words cannot hurt you. It is the hurtful things you believe about yourself, no matter where they originated, that cause you pain."

This statement was beneficial and helped me to heal old pain. I was able to feel a sense of relief and worth. Also, *up until now, and from this point forward* has changed my life. It allowed me to think change is possible, which was powerful for me.

I wrote my mother a letter but never sent it to her. There is no point because she believes that her mistreatment of me was just a form of discipline to this day. She refuses to apologize for the pain I have experienced. I truthfully feel she just did not know any better. More importantly, I wrote a letter to myself apologizing for everything I had gone through. I was able to heal what needed to be healed. Knowing that freedom is possible encouraged me to work hard. I applied Practice 9—*I practice the art of forgiveness with myself and others.* I forgive my mother. I send her love and compassion, which gives me peace. I pray for her—only God can change your heart—and have compassion for her instead of anger. I forgive myself for believing the lies for so many years. I have grown from my experience. From this point forward, I ask the challenges of my life what they are here to teach me. I will learn what needs to be learned. Healing myself from this experience has helped me release the fear that controls my mind.

* * *

I fully understand the importance of physical fitness. I walk ten thousand steps each day; I love walking. Each year for the last seven years, I have joined thousands of women and men to find a cure for cancer. I participated in a three-day walk in Chicago twice—

walking sixty miles, twenty miles each day. I now live in Canada, so I do the walk in Toronto. In the past, I walked sixty kilometers, and this year, I am signed up to walk thirty kilometers. With each kilometer I walk, I honor lives lost, including my uncle and my aunt, who I lost this year. There is not a day that goes by that I do not think about them or miss them both. Our family has never been the same without them. Even though they are not physically with me, I still feel their unbreakable spirit. I celebrate survivors, and I walk in the hope that the next generation will never experience cancer. I invite my family and friends to share this incredible journey with me by donating. Each year that I have participated, we have raised millions of dollars. This is my way of making a difference and lighting up the path to finding the cure for all cancers.

I approached inner fitness work the same way I train to walk. I need to train my mind to overcome my emotional challenges. The 14 Practices have given me the strength to shift to a positive mindset. I use them to assist me in moving from my surviving self to my thriving Self and infinite SELF. I use them as positive affirmations to overcome my greatest emotional challenges: fear, uncertainty, and anxiety. I pray each morning and night. I have the 14 Practices posted by my prayer area. I meditate on each of the practices. Every day, I set my intention for the day, depending on which one of the practices applies to my situation that day. I write it out at least ten times; I have found that the repetition helps to change and shift my mindset. As I walk with my dog Snoop, I repeat the day's practice out loud in the woods. I record it on my phone, and I listen to it during the day in my own voice, which is very powerful. In my opinion, the 14 Practices are for everyone. It does not matter who you are or what stage of life you are in.

Up till now, I had lived my life in fear, but from this point forward, I look forward to the gift of life every day brings. I know I can navigate life with different beliefs. Practice 1—*I practice turning my life over to a power greater than me.* For me that power is God, who loves me and my heart. I find so much strengthen in this practice. I am filled with God's healing power when I turn my life over to God. This has allowed me to let go of things I cannot control, including my children. "With God all things are possible" (Matthew 19:26).

I do my part with any challenges and problems I face in my life. As in Practice 2, I ask God for assistance in all I do. This practice has allowed me to sit in my observer's chair, look at what stresses me out, change what is in my control, and then ask God in prayer for his will and surrender to God, bringing my fears and worries to God's capable hands. I asked God how to free myself from the pain I feel. God sent healing in tools I received from Tina Lifford. From Practice 5—*I can choose a Self-empowering response in any situation*—I have learned that I get to choose. I have taken my power back and respond from my thriving Self because I am exhausted from just surviving. I am a great mother to my children, but I never knew I could be a great parent to myself. Practice 10—*I become a great parent and friend to myself*—has helped me treat myself better. To show my Self the same love and care I display for my children. Sometimes I write a letter as if I am giving my friend or children advice. If they were going through the same situation as me, what would I say to them? Then I take the same advice. I became the mother to myself that I always wished to have. After a trip to the store, I might come back with my favorite perfume. As I stood in the store, I saw that my favorite perfume was on sale, and I asked myself if I would buy it for my daughter. The answer was "yes," so I bought it for myself.

My wish is to have an emotionally balanced life. I am confidently moving toward living the life I dreamed of. The 14 Practices have helped me get there. I wake up excited about life and its possibilities, hoping for a better day, and trusting all mighty God. As I read my Bible, I understand more of God's words because my mindset has changed. I accept God's unconditional love. I truly believe in the inner fitness closing ritual: *I am Creative, Resilient, Empowered to choose, Whole, and Worthy.*

Being part of an Inner Fitness Circle was an incredible experience. I was surrounded by extraordinary women who were like-minded and supportive even though they had struggles of their own. It made me realize I was not alone. I looked forward to meeting with them every Monday: They inspired, empowered, and encouraged me. I shared with them openly, at a deeper level, things I have not even shared with my family. I felt safe, heard, seen, and respected. On this journey back to ourselves, we laughed together, we cried together, and we built a lifelong sisterhood. We prayed for one another, and I thank God for each one of them. Our paths have connected for a purpose. We still meet every Friday to continue this journey back to ourselves.

Alethea: Becoming Myself

MERMAIDS HAVE ALWAYS FASCINATED ME. EVER SINCE I was a girl growing up by the Atlantic Ocean, the thought of mermaids living in mystical kingdoms in the depths of the sea awakened my imagination and brought a sense of comfort. I never thought much about the mermaids' daily interactions with one another, but rather what intrigued me was how free they were, swimming and roaming about in search of mysteries and adventures. Mermaids had the ability to not worry about the dangers above the surface, and while they might have seen an occasional shark or two, they surely had a way to defend themselves from attack. This type of fantasy was exactly what I needed in my formative years, because from the time I was born and entered the world, my body was attacked.

I came out of the womb with a severe case of jaundice, and that led to many years of my parents taking me to multiple doctor appointments with no definitive answers as to the "why" behind my stunted growth, body aches, chronic vomiting, and overall malaise. It would not be discovered until my late twenties and well into my thirties that these mystery illnesses were autoimmune diseases of the colon and liver whose flare-ups would lead me down a rocky path of critical illness, brushes with death, and even a discussion of hospice that prompted me to plan my funeral just in case I didn't make it through another night.

Although these physical conditions attempted to wreak havoc, I refused to let them do so, as I made the effort to live as normally as possible under the circumstances. I had a loving family and overall support system who cared for me; I had a flourishing, award-winning career as an educator; I became a certified holistic health and wellness coach to help others view good health beyond simply diet and exercise; I participated actively in various church and sorority activities; and I made time to travel as often as possible. But, despite making the best out of unpleasant health situations, there were aspects of me beneath the surface that were unseen and unspoken—thoughts of unworthiness, a series of failed romantic relationships because I allowed myself to be carried along on a string for years, weight fluctuations, feelings of hopelessness and despair in the midst of my belief and faith, unbearable grief due to the deaths of my two best sister-friends in 2017 and 2019 from cancer, and the yearning for something *more* in life—but I had not uncovered exactly what that was.

One of the people closest to me, my older sister Dina, had more insight as to what I desired out of life, and while I couldn't quite put words to it at that time, Dina watched and listened. In fact, my sister paid such close attention that in 2020, near the beginning of the COVID pandemic, she told me of a community she had come across on social media that she thought suited my longings for that "more." She said that despite my having been in therapy and in a church small group in the past, I could learn from this online community that discussed how true evolution and change began inside through the discovery of one's true Self. The community was called the Inner Fitness Project and was led by actress Tina Lifford. When my sister sent me the Instagram link for the Inner Fitness Project,

I followed immediately and made time to see what I could glean from the posts.

Inner fitness was *different*. It went beyond the surface of who I already knew I was, and it spoke to the places I had buried and was too afraid to confront. I messaged Tina on Instagram to tell her (or her representative) how I enjoyed the posts, and she replied, inviting me to a free Wellness Wednesday session. I accepted the offer, registered, and on July 15, 2020, I attended. It was refreshing seeing women from across the nation and even in other countries share about their lives, and no one gave advice or invalidated the feelings of others. They could be themselves with no strings attached. I spoke briefly that first night, and frankly, I don't recall what I said, but I do know that I left that session more curious—yet I was afraid to take the leap fully. It would be another two years before I took the full plunge into the deep end to transform my life, and by then it was something I needed desperately.

July 20, 2022, was when I totally invested in the inner fitness community through what was known as an Inner Fitness Circle. I had just ended a relationship a month before that I knew wasn't healthy for me, and I put on a façade as if everything in my world were lovely and grand when that couldn't have been farther from the truth. I knew that during that two-year relationship I had settled for less than my worth, but because my ex-boyfriend and I had history together, I made excuses for his behavior and rationalized why I chose to hold on. I lived a lie in that relationship.

When I joined my Inner Fitness Circle, I found six incredible women who had varying experiences, yet we were there for the common goal of personal growth and a greater awareness of Self. They helped me heal from that brokenness and were a support when I needed it. Inner fitness forced me to confront my issues head-on. While I knew inner fitness wasn't therapy, it caused me to coach myself because I had no choice but to be transparent and honest about who I was and what I was deciding in my life. The inner fitness practice that resonated with me the most, and still does to this day, is Practice 11—*I tell myself the truth about what happened, my interpretation, how I feel, and what's possible.* This practice opened the door to possibilities that I had never considered.

At times it is a bit difficult for me to put into words exactly what inner fitness did for me in those first few months, but by the time I finished my Circle, I was implementing inner fitness practices daily, and they became as natural as breathing. Internal chains that held me captive for so many years were cut; the heavy loads I had carried emotionally and mentally were released; and my spirit became a mermaid in the depths of the ocean, free to roam beyond what the naked eye could see. By the end of my first year practicing inner fitness, I was active in Wellness Wednesday, and I took part in more inner fitness events, including my first Phoenix Rising workshop in early 2023. This led me to creating a vision board, and several of the goals on my vision board have already manifested a year later.

As I reflect on my journey of Self-discovery and growth through the Inner Fitness Project, I'm filled with a profound sense of gratitude and awe. Through the highs and lows, the triumphs and struggles, I've come to recognize the immense power of embracing change and my true Self, and I make daily strides toward thriving. The path of growth and evolution isn't always smooth or straightforward, for it requires vulnerability, courage, and a willingness to confront my fears and insecurities. But it has been through this process of inner fitness that I have both uncovered *and* discovered my true strength, resilience, and endless potential, which have allowed me to pursue more of my passions, dreams, and aspirations.

Self-discovery is not a destination, but a journey that has me walking in my purpose, thriving with daily joy, and being my Self authentically. As I continue this inner fitness journey, I am filled with excitement and anticipation for what the future holds. Although life comes with obstacles and setbacks, I also know both through my faith and through inner fitness that I possess the tools and the fortitude to navigate through anything, and I'm convinced that by being true to my Self and remaining open to change, I will forever be that mermaid swimming confidently, embracing the beauty of all that awaits me.

Carmen: I Lost Myself

Train up a child in the way he should go:
and when he is old, he will not depart from it.
—Proverbs 22:6

GRIEF BECAME MY STORY ON AUGUST 3, 2019—THE DAY my sister Bernadette went to live in Heaven. *Going to live in Heaven*—that phrase sounds so serene, so magical. A transcendent place where angels and ancestors reside. As she was ascending, I could not let her go.

When I lost my sister, I lost myself. I am the middle of three children. I consider it the greatest privilege that my parents raised us in a loving, faith-filled home. My mother drew from the memory of what her mother did and made us feel good about ourselves. My father showed us unconditional love up to a point. There wasn't a lot of structure in our home. We had the freedom to express ourselves, with respect. My parents also believed no child's education was complete without the incorporation of sports or artistic expression. We were involved in lots of activities and enjoyed them.

Early on, Bernadette (Bern) started developing health challenges. By the time she reached twenty-nine, her kidneys had started to fail. For twenty years, Bern was on dialysis among other challenges, such as non-Hodgkin's lymphoma. Her renal doctors often spoke about her longevity on dialysis because according to the National Kidney Foundation, the average life expectancy of a person on dialysis is five to ten years. Even more to their amazement was her positive attitude, her perseverance, and her determination to never give in or give up.

* * *

We lived life to the fullest. We traveled, had huge annual family holiday gatherings, and enjoyed movie nights and shopping extravaganzas. And through it all, not once did she complain. Even while raising her daughter, Ashley, as a single parent. Oftentimes, Ashley would sit by Bern's side at the dialysis center completing her homework assignments while her mom went through four hours of treatment, three times a week.

In June of 2019, due to long-term dialysis treatments, Bern developed cardiovascular disease, which resulted in her needing immediate open-heart surgery. The surgery was extremely complicated, and we prayed without ceasing. Her recovery was slow.

Twenty-nine days after her heart surgery, Bern suffered a massive stroke that caused severe brain damage, which required delicate brain surgery. Right now, as I type this, I have a visual of her in the cardiac critical care unit surrounded by a mountain of beeping machines *(tears)*. This led to her transition.

At that moment, it was as if a thread was pulled from me and the fabric of my life fell apart, piece by piece. I felt as if no one could help me. My family was experiencing their own grief, especially Ashley—her bond with her mother was unbreakable. My devoted husband did everything humanly possible to try and help me. I was numb.

I was empty.

I was lost.

Depression seemed to take on a life of its own. The thought of being happy again didn't play into my consciousness. It was beyond my human comprehension. Bern was my source of energy, a source of calm and reassurance. I'd surmised that life without her was purposeless. I folded up and abandoned myself for what seemed like an eternity.

* * *

You can do anything you want to do, and
you can be anything you want to be.
—Yvonne (Carmen's Mom)

Prior to losing my sister, life was good. I'd worked for twenty years for a major airline, which afforded me the luxury to travel around the world. My social circle consisted of a fun group of friends. We'd get off work on a Friday and head to Nassau for the weekend or go Christmas shopping in Paris. We had great times, but my cup wasn't full. In 2006, the airline offered an attractive "buyout" option. It was contingent upon a laundry list of factors: job performance, attendance, putting passengers first (PPF), among others. I submitted my paperwork along with hundreds of other employees and was among the fortunate selected. I left the airline with an attractive package (for life). I saw this exit as an opportunity for me to move forward with my life and embark on a new journey.

* * *

Having majored in speech communication and theater arts in college, I followed my dream and pursued a career in creative media. I studied, interned, and shadowed casting directors and producers.

My commitment and determination paid off. I became an actor and voice-over artist working in film, television, radio, and print ads. I continue working in this industry today as a member of the Screen Actors Guild and the American Federation of Television and Radio Artists (SAG-AFTRA). And in 2012, I returned to school and earned a master's degree in education.

In 2015, I became a certified women's issues and diversity trainer and a branding entrepreneur coach. With this training and my certifications, I started a small life skills business with the goal to enlighten, encourage, and empower women who were changing or starting over. Managing the business was tougher than I expected, but doing what I loved made it worth the effort. I knew that when my skills, talents, and abilities intersected, I was on my way to something beautiful, walking a path of fulfillment and purpose. Connecting with and serving others was satisfying. My bravery made me feel unstoppable. And Bern was there every step of the way.

* * *

The end of something is always the beginning of something else (the caterpillar, the chrysalis, the butterfly)
—My journal entry on 7/19/19
(as I sat next to Bern's hospital bed)

It had been a year since Bern's passing, and I was still disconnected. I knew that she wouldn't want me to live in a world of depression and grief. She wouldn't want me to abandon my purpose for thriving. Knowing this made me fully aware of the shift that was necessary for my life to return to some normality. My eureka moment came when I read *The Little Book of Big Lies*. I related to every page, every chapter, every story. "This is me!" I kept saying to myself. I wanted more.

At the end of summer 2020, I attended a Wellness Wednesday open sharing session and literally poured my heart out. I was bursting at the seams with a cry for help, and the floodgates opened and I cried endlessly that evening. I could barely utter a word. Every emotion—hurt, pain, and sorrow—revealed itself. After sharing my grief, I felt as if a weight had been lifted and like I was no longer drowning. I also experienced a light bulb moment when Tina made me aware that there is no circumstance that is bigger than me. Self-appreciation is fundamental to wellbeing, and unhappiness is fueled by a lack of Self-appreciation.

For a year, my habit of grief and depression was pulling life from me. I had abandoned my Self. For the first time, I exhaled. I pondered the thought: *Was this a window of opportunity for me to heal? Could this be the space where I could break free from my greatest emotional challenge?*

My Wellness Wednesday experience had ignited that curiosity. Afterward, I sought out inner fitness workouts as if my life depended on it. The first inner fitness workout I attended was entitled Remembering Who You Are. During the session, Tina stated, "Habits indulged become lifestyles." This statement challenged me to break free from the recurring patterns of grief and depression. Also, one of the key concepts that stood out to me was a discussion about the dominating emotions that drive our experience of the Self.

For a year, I lived in grief and depression. It was holding me back from moving forward emotionally. I enrolled in other inner fitness workouts and came away from each one with a renewed sense of possibilities for my Self. I discovered that I was getting excited about life, and I began taking steps to living fully again. I broke the habit of denying myself. I started journaling again. I was reintroduced to guided meditation, and I loved it. Following the workouts, I became part of an Inner Fitness Circle. This was a blessing—a group of women, unknown to one another, from different parts of the United States and Canada, coming together on a journey of healing and Self-rediscovery.

* * *

Within the Circle, we focused on the 14 Practices for Inner Health and Wellbeing. Every practice, every lesson, every tool was meant to be practiced outside of the Circle, to be incorporated into our daily lives. For me, the Circle also meant that God had answered a prayer as I endeavored to find inner peace and comfort—knowing that I choose to live a harmonious life.

Practice 11—*I tell myself the truth about what happened, my interpretation, how I feel, and what's possible*—became my "new story" on my inner fitness journey.

- **What happened:** My sister, my only sister, my baby sister, went to live in Heaven.
- **What I feel:** I felt like it sliced me to the bone.
- **What is possible:** Healing and happiness are possible *again*.

With Practice 14, I looked in the mirror and, once again, met the person responsible for my choices, actions, happiness, and success. Each day can bring me either joy, pain, loss, or gain.

I sat in my "observer's chair" and saw that continuing to live in grief and depression was a life imbalanced. I have the tools within me to shift, reignite my desire, and thrive again. By the end of 2020, inner fitness had become part of my life and lifestyle. I was thriving again—this time with a community on a journey to reclaim their lives as well.

In January of 2021, I participated in another inner fitness workout series called Phoenix Rising. A-M-A-Z-I-N-G!!!

My experience of Phoenix Rising is summarized in a lyrical expression piece that I wrote:

METAMORPHOSIS

Just as a baby bird raises its head to sing the dawn of a new day
I sing of endless *possibilities* as I *shift* on this journey underway.

Just as a butterfly emerges from its broken skin
So has my soul from the shell and confinement of grief within.

Just as a baby sings its first cry, born from a mother's womb
I am a rebirth, from pain to power; here I stand, in full bloom.

Up until now, grief became my *sacred torture* of imprisonment
But from this point forward, I'm the dragonfly, *fully alive* and
    present.

I *SWOOSH*, preparing an atmosphere for my *Self's* destiny
For it is there that I *thrive*, walking in truth to my *infinity*.

I really love who I'm becoming, I love how I'm *ascending*.
I dance freedom within this *metamorphosis* of my being.

Escaping the flames of *big lies*
From a pile of ashes, *LIKE A PHEONIX, I RISE!*

Most importantly, inner fitness has helped me realize that my
allegiance to my sister Bernadette means that I will continue to
walk in my truth as I know she would want me to. And God will
honor that.

Deidre: I Was My Achievements

I AM A NATIVE OF DENVER, COLORADO. A SINGLE MOTHER OF two young adult sons, I have always considered myself a lifelong learner. Joining the Inner Fitness Project community has provided me with something I never knew I was missing—the language, tools, and self-compassion to finally focus my passion for learning on myself and on my relationship with myself. This has been a gift.

In 2014 my father died after an eighteen-month battle with undiagnosed dementia. I was a Daddy's Girl, so the loss of the parent who had been such a nurturing, demanding force of nature was life-altering. Within three months of his death, I was laid off from my job at a foundation. The layoff caused an unexpected jolt to my longtime role as the sole provider for my family. Within a few months, I finally decided to get divorced and extract myself from a failing and harmful marriage. During the divorce process, I had to get a restraining order. For a while my life felt like a reality show that I would never want to watch. I used to joke with close friends that my life had exploded, and I was about the business of reimagining and reassembling myself. The focus of that self-development work was how to be the best single mother I could be and how to be an effective leader. Through it all, I stayed on autopilot, dutifully showing up for each of my many roles.

I am also the CEO and executive director of a community-based public health nonprofit. During the height of the COVID-19 pandemic, we worked to provide essential services and supplies throughout our metro area, navigating so much need while not taking the time to personally process so much community loss. I spent my days reviewing virus statistics and participating in discussions regarding ethical strategies to determine who would live and who would be denied access to early medications. Once vaccines were finally available, I was fighting for equitable access. Personally, in an eighteen-month period, I lost four cousins (three within a single week in April 2020), two uncles, and three aunts. Looking back, I didn't truly take time to grieve for any of them. I did not know how to with everything I had on my plate. I just kept working.

In late 2021, when I saw the online ad for a Phoenix Rising workshop to begin in 2022, I immediately signed up. In addition to being familiar with Tina Lifford from her acting career, I had already purchased her first book after hearing her speak at a Women Creating Our Futures conference in Denver in January 2020. When I signed up for that first Phoenix Rising workshop, I had already done some great work on managing the external aspects of my life. I had moved my sons into a beautiful new home and focused on being the best mother I could be without a co-parent or any financial support. Life already felt easier with just the three of us. In a short period of time, I had also transformed the nonprofit. I had changed the business model, tripled the budget, and purchased a building. I viewed having an ongoing baseline of stress as simply a symptom of being a Black woman in America. Now I can say that despite the external successes, I did not have a relationship with myself—beyond pushing myself to the limit to prove my worth and accomplishments.

I inadvertently came to my healing journey via a leadership development path. I was raised to believe that my value was based on my accomplishments and to take pride in achievements. I attended Princeton and Yale, two environments that only amplified the emphasis on achievement. Throughout my career I continued to view my worthiness through the lens of my accomplishments. The year after my divorce I was invited to apply for and was accepted into three significant leadership fellowships. My surviving self kept saying "Yes!" believing that this was life flooding in after my course correction of a divorce and that these simultaneous opportunities were rewards for my previous hard work. Which makes sense in navigating a leadership journey. After the challenges of the pandemic, my surviving self became a confident pro at spur-of-the-moment interviews and speaking engagements. I frequently shared with other women leaders the importance of standing in your truth and knowing your own worth. But what I now realize is that I understood my worth only in relation to others.

It wasn't until I began my Inner Fitness Project journey that I was able to discern that my compulsive need to stay busy was not an exhausting byproduct of success, but was rooted in the belief that my worth was based on what I had achieved or what I was doing for others.

I have had two executive coaches in the past as well as three fellowships that all have touched on the importance of self-knowledge and development in the context of a leadership journey. While my leadership training opportunities truly supported my personal and professional growth, the focus was always the end goal of being able to identify and capitalize on my leadership strengths. I am grateful for those local and national opportunities, which helped me hone my communication skills, understand executive presence, and learn how to articulate my ideas with clarity in order to have a positive influence in the world. But while valuable, all those things are based on external relationships.

I now understand that it is really easy to celebrate those types of successes and still, often unknowingly, neglect the most important relationship—the one we have with our Selves.

The emphasis of leadership training is on decision-making and problem-solving—things at which I have always excelled. So, when I was able to navigate complex situations with confidence, when I could assess and analyze team dynamics in real time, it was easy to convince myself that those tangible self-development benefits were also positively showing up in other aspects of my life. And that was partially true for external relationships. I also had some success with an emotion integration coach, where I learned that it is truly impossible to compartmentalize my personal and professional selves. With every new tool I was given, I was always quick to pivot or adjust. I enjoyed receiving positive feedback: "Deidre, you are so responsible and responsive." Yet, I rarely shared that I tackled these assignments and tasks as I would anything else: to get an A+, to complete the assignment.

It wasn't until I joined the Inner Fitness Project community that I was finally able to apply a very clear model that resonated with me and allowed me to see my Three Selves. To understand that even though I had been on my healing journey, I had been tackling the easy stuff. It was superficial, external, and limited because my surviving self was in control and in the lead, taking care of business when it came to what healing could look like for me. If I wanted to keep going, I would have to *get curious* about me.

In addition to a framework that can be effectively applied daily, the Inner Fitness Project provides a peer group of other individuals on a similar personal journey. There is always a warm welcome in every meeting, whether virtual or in-person.

Today I embrace all of me—while I am still trying to practice slowing down. The more time I spend working on my relationship with myself and being curious about my surviving self, thriving Self, and infinite SELF, the more ease I experience, and the less anxiety. I also know that these changes are reflecting in my external personal and professional relationships—as a mother, daughter, sister, CEO, board member, and friend. With each new year of the Inner Fitness Project, I can reflect on how far I have come and still be more and more curious about myself and practice releasing any judgment of myself or others. I now understand that if I do not mourn the past, I can't envision the future. Now that I have a relationship with myself, I have started processing those losses that I have left unaddressed for so long. Up until now, I had to prove I was worthy on a daily basis. As Tina Lifford reminds us, we have the power and right to choose, and choose, again and again.

I choose me.

Elizabeth: My Corporate Fall

IN THE SUMMER OF 2013, I WAS AT THE TOP OF MY CAREER game when I received an offer to oversee a pretty big corporate team with a large financial obligation. Around that time, I'd spent more than two decades in the corporate sector—an environment where, with just a high school diploma, I'd worked my way up from secretarial positions to leading high-profile businesses. Promotion after promotion, I hungered for more.

Before the offer, I had worked on a special project that landed in the business section of the *New York Times*. Confident that my years of experience would drive this new team to success, I accepted the role as a senior director and hit the ground running.

Not long after starting my new position, I found myself struggling to get support from my peers to do my job. When I introduced myself as the new member of the team and went to shake a hand, I was met with, "I don't shake hands." When I shared my brand and product strategies, my vision was frowned upon. When I walked into meetings, I was ignored. When I accomplished the goals I set, instead of hearing "good job," I heard about flaws in the project. Nonetheless, I kept going. I even went as far as carrying limited-edition designer handbags into meetings to get a reaction from my peers, knowing they were designer junkies, too. But nothing.

After a while, my efforts to be accepted in this new environment began to take a toll on me. My confidence suddenly was overshadowed by self-doubt. I'll never forget the day I had an emotional breakdown at work. The single-breasted black blazer I wore was adorned with a black-and-white striped floral pin that sat on my left lapel. The olive-drab silk joggers gathered perfectly around my waist, covering my graphic T-shirt. And the black leather peep-toe ankle booties pulled the entire athleisure look together according to the fashion trends at the time. When I stopped to gaze at my reflection in the floor-to-ceiling mirror, I admired the outfit and audibly said, "You look cute today!" And just as soon as the word *today* rolled off my tongue, the imperceptible thought that followed was *But you are all fucked up inside*. I remember walking fast from the bathroom to my office and quickly closing the door, sobbing uncontrollably. *Maybe my peers are right*, I said to myself. The unyielding persona I'd always displayed in the workplace was slowly drifting away.

Before long, going into the office became a challenge. My nights were restless. During the day, my energy was low. I was mentally and emotionally depleted. One mental health day became two mental health days, which then turned into three mental health days. I'd missed three straight days of work and had been in bed with the blinds closed for the fourth straight day. I had not eaten much during that time. Self-judgment played on a constant loop in my head and would not shut up. I tried sleeping to escape the noise. When sleep refused to come, I'd curl up in a ball and weep. On day three of missing work, my boss called to check on me. I assured her I was okay and I would be back in the office the next day to prepare for an upcoming business trip. But I was not okay.

Lying in bed, crippled by my emotions, was not just about the challenges I faced at work. Midway into this new role, I had met a man. For two decades, I'd unconsciously shielded my heart from being broken. Suddenly, I had the courage to conquer my fears and opened myself up to a long-distance relationship.

It was a mutual attraction after just one meeting. The texting, the calls, the compliments, and the praise from afar felt familiar—yet unfamiliar. And the more attention I received, the more I craved. Any time of the day, any hour of the night, I made myself available when I heard from him. On occasion, we'd talk for hours. I wanted to share with him every move I made. But after a while, he did not want to do the same with me. Whenever I experienced a lull in our communication, I obsessed over what I had done wrong or whether I had said something to upset him. I found myself apologizing when I had nothing to apologize for. I didn't recognize the submissive person I had become after falling fast and hard for this stranger.

A month later, I attended my first psychotherapy session. I knew if I didn't get professional help quickly, I could lose my job, my home, and more important at the time, my image. I went into therapy thinking I would deal with my intimacy issues and maybe talk about my struggles at work. I soon discovered that neither was the problem. Both experiences, however, had triggered unresolved childhood trauma. Trauma I'd unconsciously kept at bay for forty years.

When I was eight years old, I moved from New York to North Carolina to live with my grandmother. For the next eighteen months while I was there, I convinced myself that my mother didn't want or love me. I fantasized about the father I didn't know and pretended he would rescue me. I believed the only way to gain their love and attention was to be perfect. Because if I was perfect, then I would be praised. When praised, I felt loved. Feeling loved gave me a sense of belonging. And if I belonged, I must be good enough. If I am good enough, I won't be abandoned or rejected ever again.

I unconsciously carried this vicious cycle of beliefs from childhood into adulthood. They informed my behavior and the relationship choices I made along my journey. Chasing perfectionism is what sent me on a path to seek external validation from things and people to prove my worth. Chasing perfectionism is also what brought me to my knees and forced me to confront my trauma.

At work, the limited-edition designer handbags I thought would save me in meetings were just my way of masking the underlying pain I had experienced as a child whenever I felt rejected by my peers. The valuable lesson that I learned, but took time for me to grasp, is that my worth isn't measured by my work.

As for the relationship, on the days when that man felt withdrawn, cold, and emotionally unavailable, he showed up as my distant mother. On days he showered me with attention, compliments, and love, he was the father I yearned for. It would be some time before I was able to let him go, even knowing he was mostly a catalyst to teach me that I didn't love myself.

Learning to love and honor myself was an arduous struggle. Years of therapy provided me with tools not only to care for myself, but to mother the eight-year-old in me. She needed healing, too. She needed to know she did nothing wrong. She needed love. And the more I loved on her, the more compassion and forgiveness I developed for myself and for the choices my mother had made to mother me the way she did. Over time, I changed the narrative about my father, too. For years, I had placed him on a pedestal. But the truth is, he was never present in my life.

Up until my self-discoveries in therapy, I was attached to my looks, my career, my money, my title, my relationships, and my lavish vacations. I lived a life of fantasy. If I looked good on the outside, no one would see the hurt and pain destroying me on the inside. Not even me. Now I am just as comfortable rocking sweatpants as I am wearing a designer suit. I carry a handbag with no visible logo to a part-time retail job that fulfills me in different ways. Joy comes to me when I throw a spontaneous party for one and dance alone. I practice gratitude daily and meditate often. I have learned to say "no" to protect my inner peace. I say "yes" when I'm offered love from others because I now believe I deserve love, especially the love I give myself.

Fast-forward to 2021, when I found myself falling into old patterns and beliefs. The COVID pandemic had taken a toll on my mental and spiritual psyche. By midyear, I'd sunk into a depressive state again. That summer, I had the opportunity to join the Inner Fitness Project with seven Black women: strangers. For fourteen weeks, we Zoomed and shared and cried and laughed together. We discussed our personal struggles and how to use the 14 Practices offered by Tina Lifford to grow in sovereignty. I go back to the root cause of my pain and echo Practice 4—*I look for and work to transform the beliefs, patterns, and judgments I practice that limit my life.* All the wisdom I gained in the Inner Fitness Project reinforced my learnings in therapy. I'm grateful to have both as part of my healing journey.

Freida: Finding My Truth

I HAD BEEN LIVING MY ADULT LIFE WITH A SMILE ON MY face and a lie in my heart.

I created a professional career as an entrepreneur. I had reached a financial status that allowed me to care for my loved ones, my daughter, and myself. I gave to strangers in need and, I thought, nurtured myself. I say "thought" because I purchased "things" for myself as a way of taking care of myself.

I lost my mother in 1997 and my sister after a three-year battle with cancer in 2010. It was the year everything—every movement, every word, every deed—seemed to hurt with a pain so deep that, at times, I would leave the office, drive past my home, and just continue driving, listening to CDs my sister had loaded before her death, and crying until there were no more tears for the day. I would then go home, greet my husband, and wish I could disappear.

I made awful financial and personal decisions, and prayed for my head to stop pounding and for my heart to stop beating with sadness. My sister was my friend. We did everything together; our relationship was unwavering on my part. I felt her pain and watched her grow professionally. I watched her draw on her faith and continue to "buy" love while continually trying to shower her with love, time, gifts, and understanding. NO judgment. I understood her as

I had observed her pain as a child. I felt guilty as everything always seemed easier for me. Lie number one! Life had never been easy for me, *never*!

I felt obligated to my mother and siblings to be *the one* who could and would *fix* everything for everyone. I was considered the uncontrollable, crazy, wild, brilliant one. The child who did not need to be comforted, who everyone could turn to and rely on in hard times. I was the one who made everything better. Before I was old enough to earn money to fix matters, I ran errands, cleaned the house, did laundry, and defended my mother in episodic moments that I should not have even been aware of at my age.

My parents were married for twenty-three years, and for the first five years, my mother worked and went through fertility treatments. She wanted not just to have a child, she wanted ten children. After my father completed college in Chicago, my parents moved back to a small Midwestern town, where her continued fertility treatments *worked*! She became pregnant with me. Both of my parents were overjoyed, as were their siblings and parents. The loving couple was now going to be complete. I was born on February 28, according to my mother, or on February 29 at 4:00 a.m., according to her older sister. I listened to this disagreement off and on my entire childhood, and I'm pretty sure my aunt is correct. I mention this tidbit to illustrate how any and everything my mother said I defended, from small matters to extremely obviously wrong, hurtful matters.

It all started as my mother shared her childhood journey with me while I was still technically a child. Hence, I spent my entire life, even when angry with her, feeling compassion and a sense that I had to make her life better.

She lost her mother when she was seven years old, and her mother's family convinced her father that he was not capable of raising an incorrigible (and brilliant) little girl. From that point on, her version of events is that she was sent from relative to relative and called crazy.

By the time I was nine years old, my loving father had turned into a verbally, emotionally, and physically abusive husband. I understand today what caused his "new" behavior. However, to this day I find it abhorrent.

I also loved him. I was almost seventeen when she divorced him. However, that was not the end of their story. They died two years apart—Dad first, then Mother. She grieved her loss despite having spent twenty-three years living with her new partner and doing life as she now saw fit. At twenty-three, I married my daughter's father, who was close to a duplicate of my abusive father. I divorced him when she was two years old, and I will live with the scars, physical and emotional, for the rest of my life. I decided he was not under any circumstances going to stunt my growth as a mother, daughter, professional, or woman. At twenty-five, I set out to conquer the world and become the best loving role model I could be for my beautiful, deserving daughter.

No man would ever have my heart trapped in madness and strip me of my confidence. I went to therapy to address what I had endured during the marriage. When the therapist tried to get to the root of my issues, we had one session with my mother. I never went back to that therapist.

My mother called my siblings and her siblings to express how hurt she was with what I had to say about her and to talk about how she had given her life to her children. I was an ungrateful person that would pay for saying negative things about her to the therapist.

I was devastated.

I was lectured for weeks by two aunts about how the Bible states, "Honor thy father and thy mother." I cried myself to sleep after putting my daughter to bed and asked God to forgive me. I should have just kept those feelings to myself. Lie number two!

* * *

From that point on until her death, I dedicated myself to her every whim or need. I made financial plans to position myself to take care of my daughter's needs and to provide for myself as a senior. I never wanted to ask my daughter for anything or make her feel the guilt I felt over my mother's life and bad decisions.

I moved from the Midwest to the West Coast to start anew. Still, the miles between us did not stop the monetary commitments, nor did the move give me the strength to say "no." I watched all my investments dwindle and eventually disappear altogether, but forced myself to believe I had made the "right" move.

The six years between my sister's death and the night I acknowledged the lies were the most excruciating of my life.

* * *

One night, I had the pleasure of listening to Tina Lifford read a couple of chapters from *The Little Book of Big Lies*. She had chosen three or four people to email chapters and get their feedback. I asked her to read chapters aloud. This happened for about a month, and I was engrossed in her Inner Fitness Project.

I found myself thinking about the words and concepts, and what grabbed me the most was—and remains—the importance of acknowledging the lies. At one in the morning, in the middle of a chapter Tina was reading, I broke down and began sobbing uncontrollably. I apologized to Tina, and she immediately responded, "No apology needed, my dear Freida. It has been a long time coming!"

She then asked, "What are you thinking and what are you feeling?"

I said, "Tina, I knew they were lies; I knew why I kept burying them deeper and deeper into my soul and my heart; it was my continued effort to protect everyone except myself. The little girl inside me so needed to play. I have manipulated therapists for decades. I resumed therapy after my initial disastrous session in another state, with therapists who did not know anything about my life, my mother, my daughters, my siblings, or my struggles. Always my relationships with therapists became more friendly than therapeutic, and two of them asked me to go into practice with them. I declined; I liked working alone, being alone. Funny if you saw me 'work' a room, you would never guess how comfortable I am with alone."

I believe that night God intervened and placed Tina and the Inner Fitness Project into my life and my heart. I have continued to study. I have navigated through the mishmash of lies and allowed the little girl in me to come out and play. I graduated from living in my "surviving self" to wrapping my life around my thriving Self. My smile is now genuine, and I don't need anyone in the room to show me joy. Why? Because Inner Fitness has taught me that "I am enough!"

I shared my thoughts, my reality, with Tina. God placed the Inner Fitness Project in my life when he knew I would need it the most. The following year, after I had begun a serious daily inner fitness practice, I was diagnosed with stage 4 non-small cell cancer of the lungs. I had surgery, and according to the surgeon, with treatment I would live no more than six months. That was ten years ago. This past May, I suffered two massive heart attacks, and two months later I lost the use of my right leg due to damage to my peripheral nerve.

Today, I walk independently with the use of both legs. The cancer is stable, and the medical team has removed me from some of the heart medication. Life is not perfect, but there is no doubt that had

I been living with the burden of "the lies" and not doing the work, I would not have had the strength to endure and come through the challenges I have faced.

It is my personal belief that we are all given a task by whatever higher power you believe in—our purpose. We must be still to understand and follow commands, and we don't all do that either. Yet when we do, when we allow ourselves to become a vessel, the truth, the facts, the creations, and the inventions come to those chosen for the task.

I thank God that he chose to use Tina as the vessel to spread the word, work, and tools of her Inner Fitness Project. It takes so much that many never see to disseminate the teaching, yet the load is much lighter when you live the word you teach.

I implore those in silent pain, living the big lie, to "put your armor on." It's tailor-made to your very own perfect size. You will find strength and joy you did not know possible, right inside the words of and training offered through the Inner Fitness Project.

Jacquie: Heart Palpitations

P RACTICE 4—*I LOOK FOR AND WORK TO TRANSFORM THE beliefs, patterns, and judgments I practice that limit my life*—is transformational for me. It is the undergirding of my truth that fuels my desire as it points me toward my more authentic life.

My mantra for living has been Romans 12:2: "Do not be conformed to the patterns of this world, but be transformed by the renewing of your mind." Practice 4 has allowed this mantra to come to life in my life.

March 21, 2019, I was lying in an emergency room with a doctor telling me that my blood enzyme levels indicated I had experienced a heart attack in the previous twenty-four hours. I had thought I was just sick with the flu, with weakness and dizzy spells. But my daughter insisted I go to the hospital. By the time I got out to the car, I was having trouble walking, and my left shoulder and arm were tingling.

I ended up being in the hospital for two weeks, getting an angiogram, having every kind of test possible, and being referred to specialists. I was diagnosed with supraventricular tachycardia, or SVT, a type of irregular heartbeat. It was not a heart attack. But I was assigned a cardiologist, who coordinated my health care with my general practitioner, endocrinologist, and cardiac surgeon. I also brought to my health-care team a therapist and someone who specialized in health behavior medical psychotherapy. I was a mess.

I spent much of my life as an overworking perfectionist who was reactive and lived a fear-based lifestyle. After getting married and having four children, I didn't make any time for myself. I came from a household that taught me to keep busy and work my butt off at all costs. I was taught to deny any "selfish" thought of doing anything for myself.

After that hospital experience, the next two years of my life ended up being a turning point. I started to prioritize my physical health. I learned that the heart palpitations that I had been experiencing for forty years were my body talking to me, telling me that it needed attention. For the first time I also focused on my mental health, learning about listening to my body and uncovering the gem of my spiritual self. There was stigma attached to seeking mental wellness in my family, so I hadn't realized it was something that a person could ever need.

In June 2020, one of my favorite spiritual teachers, Michael Beckwith, mentioned a book called *The Little Book of Big Lies*. That day I buried myself in YouTube videos and got to know the author, Tina Lifford. I had this bizarre feeling that she knew me, and her spirit vibrated with mine. I bought the audiobook the same day.

Halfway through the first chapter, I called my sister-friend and told her that she *had* to get this book. This was the start of my inner fitness journey.

I had spent more than forty years dabbling in positive mental attitude (PMA) books and resources. Nothing hit my soul like this amazing book, which kept me following a recipe for success that was practical and consistent. My sister-friend was just as excited as I was, and we started attending Wellness Wednesdays, as well as following other social media and inner fitness sessions.

I started attending a weekly Inner Fitness Circle with nine other inner fitness community members. Part of our sessions included focusing on one of the 14 Practices each week. Practice 4—*I look for and work to transform the beliefs, patterns, and judgments I practice that limit my life*—was mine. I felt as though Tina wrote it just for me. Up until that point I had been shaped by fear and doing everything I could to please and help everyone else, to my own detriment.

In my life I embraced God's word as tight as I embraced all my fears. Fear motivated my prayers, dictated my spiritual life, and buried the mustard seed far away from my reach. I was in rough spiritual shape. I believed that the ebb and flow of words that came at me needed my approval, reaction, and judgment. This created sickness in my body, soul, and spirit. I knew that God's infinite spirit was inside of me, but I got lost in the religion of the Christian faith sifting through sermons, penned representations, and other people's definitions of what the true faith was. God's word was not living in me; it was marred by the filter of society that I thought was my truth.

The Little Book of Big Lies was like God tapping on my shoulder saying, *Pay attention, Jacquie; look deep.*

Practice 4 woke me up. It shook religion off me and pointed me directly to my relationship with my infinite SELF, which was hiding within me. There was the thing that I was missing in Romans 12:2—"Do not be conformed to the patterns of this world, but be transformed by the renewing of your mind"; the word *renewing* is a present participle. It is a process of shedding the old outer covering and putting on the new. I realized that to transform the beliefs, patterns, and judgments that I practiced, I needed to continuously lean in, observe, and adjust. I had to do the work.

So now with Practice 4 in mind, from this point forward I get curious and ask myself questions about the lies that I had believed up until now. I depend on God's infinite spirit to point me to old patterns that limit my life. I put judgment aside and know that I am learning to control my thoughts. I am also practicing making my mind a servant through daily prayer, meditation, and reflection. I am willing to let go of behaviors that no longer serve me because I am focused on living each moment as it shows up and choosing my responses. This is where the shift started happening.

The ongoing practice of looking for beliefs, patterns, and judgments has continued to pull me along. I created a beautiful prayer wall and reflection area that inspires me each day. I have been observing my reactions and choosing my responses after careful reflection and sometimes a deep, cleansing breath. I have discovered that I love being me. I truly do love myself, and I have certainly incorporated into my life Practice 1—*I practice turning my life over to a power greater than me that loves me and responds to my heart.*

I know that my health issue in 2019 was a *gift* that God gave me to wake me up and get my attention. I am so thankful for this gift, and each day I am excited when my eyes open in the morning and I send out appreciation to God for being alive. I see my future as an open opportunity to choose. I recognize that I need to focus on Practice 10—*I become a great parent and friend to myself*—because I need to always take care of myself and my spirit. I also recognize that my vibration is attracting different things to my life now that I'm paying attention. In November 2020, I found out about a newly created position with my former employer. I was not looking for a new job, but one thing led to another and I ended up getting that job. I believe my new vibration attracted this position to me because I was ready.

Each week that I attend my Inner Fitness Circle and choose one of the 14 Practices to work with, I feel as though the practice dictates my week because it shows up for me and I am looking for it. Each practice has allowed me to continue my journey to *renew my mind* each day. I have grown to realize that my life is challenging, but now I am continuously observing, shifting, and choosing. My new awakening takes daily practice; it is not easy, because sometimes old habits call my name. This is when I must forgive myself and appreciate better choices for the future. I believe that I'm up for the challenge, but I don't want to fool myself into thinking that I can do it on my own. My Inner Fitness Circle is so important to me. I have found nine sisters and a community that have allowed me to show up as myself. They get me. They have journeyed with me and hugged me and cried with me. In my house, my family members know that Wellness Wednesday is my weekly event and I'm committed to being there and showing up for myself.

I often consider how I got to a point in my life where I was totally disconnected from my soul and forgot about my Self. I believe that low self-esteem has been my primary issue. I think back to the time when I was a small child in elementary school and the children called me *blackie Jacquie.* Or when I was in eighth grade, a week away from graduation, and my teacher called me over and said, "I will not be graduating you because I don't have to pass all of *your kind.*" I believed the lies that told me I wasn't good enough and that to get through life I had to always have a smile on my face no matter how I was treated or how I was feeling. I was surrounded by negative ideas about people who looked like me, so I went out of my way to prove that I wasn't what other people assumed I was. Amid all these things, I lost myself. I looked at the way I saw my mother demonstrating her role, and I assumed that was exactly what I needed to do as well. It took getting sick for me to hit my lowest point and come back to my Self.

I am a strong, beautiful child of God. I love me and I love being me. I use daily affirmations to recognize how amazing I am. This is the important way that I have found to nourish my soul and renew my mind. I lean in and listen to my spirit. It is God-given and knows what is good for me. I meditate every day and continuously pray to God, as he is my source and his Holy Spirit lives in me. I feel healthy and I know that my surviving self would like nothing better than to take over again. To maintain my health and welfare, I must continue to renew my mind. This inner fitness journey is how I love my Self. I am so thankful to have the 14 Practices to help me navigate and continue to challenge me to be selfish (in a healthy way).

My relationships are now deeper and much healthier. I recognize that change begins with me, and I have rediscovered how getting to know myself has freed me from the shackles of oppression. I remember getting some advice when I was young: *You can use your money to buy pretty stuff that will temporarily satisfy you. But buying a good book will open your mind to endless possibilities and perspectives that will expand your thinking and beliefs. Invest in yourself.*

Recently I visited my optometrist to get my annual eye exam. As per usual, it consisted of a series of lenses being presented to me and the repeated question: "Which is better, 1 or 2?" and so on. At the end of the exam the optometrist showed me the difference between my current lenses and the up-to-date prescription that I would need to fill. It was remarkably different, even though she said there was only a slight adjustment to the prescription, both for my distance and for my reading lenses.

This made me think of the Inner Fitness Workouts and being part of the inner fitness community. Each workout provides me with incremental adjustments to help me to progress through life as it presents itself. During the workouts I don't always realize the impact of the exercises. But I continue to do them as I have faith that they will have long-term impacts. Since I know that I am worth the investment as a precious child of a King, I will continue my inner fitness journey as part of my newly incorporated lifestyle.

Kia: Daddy's Girl

———

A S I AM SITTING DOWN TO WRITE THIS, IT'S THE DAY AF-
ter what would have been my father's seventy-sixth birthday;
he died a little over a year and a half ago at the age of seventy-four.
When I was a child, you never could have convinced me that I
would be standing after the loss of my parents. Yet, here I am, and
I owe it to inner fitness; I owe it to leaning in to the 14 Practices; I
owe it to a new perspective, the ability to look at life one moment
at a time. I owe it to my newfound awareness that the practice of
inner fitness will be something I need for the rest of my life because
as surely as I breathe, life will continue to show up and do what life
does. Get bumpy.

I am the child of two amazingly flawed humans. I was born and
raised by high school sweethearts. I had a wonderful childhood;
my parents worked hard to give me opportunities they didn't have.
It was beautiful, but just like anything else, our lives had ups and
downs. My dad was my superhero; in my eyes, there was nothing
he couldn't do. He was often the most remarkable person in the
room, the social butterfly; my mom was caring, reserved, and someone everyone leaned on. She would rather stay home on a Friday
night, but he couldn't wait to attend any function. Yet somehow,
they worked.

Reflecting on life with my parents, I see glaring examples of both the need for inner fitness and times when inner fitness was alive and well. My mom carried the world's weight on her shoulders, often taking care of everyone but herself, and my dad sometimes ran away from problems by pretending they didn't exist. When I was a kid, we lived in an apartment. I remember two things about that apartment: the kitchen, and watching my mom do everything a mom would do, including making my birthday cakes and my favorite treat, Jell-O. And fires—there were always fires; the alarm would go off, and my parents would throw a coat over my head and hold me close as they carried me down the six flights of stairs out of the building.

Between constant fires and deteriorating living conditions, my mom wanted more for us; she wanted to own a home. She was scared and had no idea how she would make it happen, but despite her fears and limiting beliefs, she did it anyway. Through inner fitness I've learned "if you can see it, you can change it," and looking back, I see that this might be the first instance I remember of that at play in my mom's life. She said we were getting a house even though my dad questioned how we could afford it. But she never wavered and trusted that what was in her heart would prevail.

When inner fitness found me, I was forty eight years old. I had lived through my dad's drug addiction and recovery. He was the best human I and many others knew, yet he struggled with addiction. He struggled with life bumping into life, layoffs from his work, and the death of his brother. If he had had inner fitness tools, he might have avoided addiction. I didn't see his addiction until I was out of college, although there were signs. Recreation met up with life, and at some point, he lost control of it—no longer able to go to work, function, and be the husband and dad we all knew and loved. But at the time of his death, he had more than twenty-five years of sobriety.

When inner fitness found me, I had transitioned from corporate America to being an entrepreneur, from the security of knowing when my next paycheck was coming to operating without a safety net. I had lived through two cancer diagnoses, the first being ovarian cancer at the age of thirty-three, three weeks before my first wedding anniversary. I went through eight rounds of chemotherapy and had a total hysterectomy, which left me incapable of having children of my own. Years later I was diagnosed with early-stage breast cancer, which resulted in a double mastectomy. I had become a mom unconventionally. I had lived through the death of my mom, my best friend, and I did not know it then, but I was preparing to say goodbye to my first love, my dad, six months after starting my inner fitness journey.

The universe knows what you need; I believe that with everything I am. I had been attending the Inner Fitness Project's Wellness Wednesdays consistently for about six months before my dad entered hospice. I never mentioned his illness during our time of noncompulsory sharing; I couldn't. I was doing everything I could to will him into optimal health, and let's be honest—I knew I would never make it through that share without ugly crying. It turns out I couldn't outrun my dad's illness, ultimate prognosis, and the Wellness Wednesday share that needed to happen. My dad had been in hospice care for a couple of days. While tending to him during his final days with us, my husband suggested I not skip Wellness Wednesday. He had seen proof of the work I was putting in on my inner wellness, and he thought now was the time to lean in. I signed on to the virtual meeting, left my camera off, and proceeded to share through inaudible tears that my father was dying. I knew I wouldn't make it through the share without crying, but at that point, I was so full of pain I needed a safe place to say I was sad and scared, and that one of my biggest fears (up until that point) was coming true:

the death of my dad. My favorite human was transitioning; after my mom had passed nine years before, he became both parents to me. He was everything I needed him to be and never took his foot off the gas after my mom passed. So there I sat, crying my eyes out to a room of people I had "known" for only a few months, but it didn't matter; that was the share I needed. I needed to get that out; I needed to be honest; I needed to tell myself the truth. My dad was dying. It didn't make his passing painless, but it gave me the strength to walk beside him with complete vulnerability and no regrets.

As Tina says, life will bump into life, and just like clockwork, life showed up again. This time, five months after my dad's passing, my grandmother, my father's mother, passed at the age of 101. My journey to becoming practiced through inner fitness allowed me to show up for my grandmother in ways I never imagined. She wasn't the same after my dad passed; she often expressed that it was "no longer fun" to be here. Being on the journey of inner fitness helped me to make peace with the impending loss of my grandmother. I could choose how to respond to her final months, weeks, and days. I cried and cried, but I also loved and loved. I enjoyed every moment with her; I made her laugh, she made me laugh, I sat with her, I napped with her, and I told her I loved her repeatedly. I didn't blame God or the universe; I didn't ask "Why us?" The old me would have been so angry because we had just lost my dad. Instead, I said, *I'll miss her terribly, but how lucky are we to have had her for 101 years?* How lucky am I to have known her as an adult? It's a special gift to know your grandparents as an adult. My maternal grandmother died when I was just nineteen. My paternal grandmother died seven days before my forty-ninth birthday, and her funeral was on my birthday. My newish understanding that life will continue to show up, bump into life, and create more life allowed me to see that this moment was my grandmother's final gift. When would I ever have a chance to have my entire family in one place on my birthday? We celebrated a life that was and a life that is, simultaneously, because two things can be true. We can be sad that life is over and rejoice at the gift of another trip around the sun.

If you look at my bookshelf, I have enough self-help books to last me a lifetime. I have read many of them in their entirety, and started and stopped many of them because they just didn't click. I pride myself on resilience; I have been through a lot and am still here. I have sat with Buddhist monks in Thailand to learn about mindset. I thought I was well-practiced, but I now realize I was holding my breath until I could get to the other side of whatever the mountain of life had placed in front of me. I am great at being re-silient after a storm has passed. When I knew for sure that I would survive my ovarian cancer diagnosis, I became an advocate. I spoke to nursing students, started a blog, and shared my story whenever I could. I made my mess my message, as they say. I did it when it was safe to do so. I didn't realize then that I was waiting for permission to live, but looking back, that's what I was doing.

My daughter came into my life when she was four. I loved her from a distance until I knew it was safe to love her without fear of losing her. What would my journey have been like if I had the tools of inner fitness years ago? I wouldn't have pushed past adversity; I might have seen my situation as it is, with no judgment, made empowering choices, and alleviated some of the turmoil and pain that goes with figuring out how to move forward. I had no choice but to go toward fear and adversity, but the ride would have been smoother. I thought I had a handle on life, but I was just touching the surface. Through inner fitness, I am learning that every experience has been for my greater good. I am who I am because of each of these experiences. I can honestly say I am having the time of my life in one of the most challenging chapters in my book. I am having a better time than when I thought life couldn't get any better. The difference is that I am now aware, awake, engaging, and *thriving*.

Krista: Grief and Change

1999

April 9 was devastating. It was the day my sister passed away in a Los Angeles hospital, and my life began to unravel.

As I sat with my family outside of her room a few minutes after her death, I couldn't bear the sound of sobs and the smell of the hospital another minute. Without saying a word, I got up and walked out for some space, fresh air, and perspective.

I wandered around the parking lot for several minutes before plopping down on a distant curb. I cried out, "Oh God, I wish I were anywhere but here! I wish I were on top of a mountain!"

Immediately, I wondered about that bizarre request. I had never climbed a mountain. But in that heart-wrenching moment, I had a vision of myself sitting on top of a grassy mountaintop.

Two weeks later, I did something I'd never done: I booked an appointment with a spiritual counselor. I had never heard of this counselor before, but something inside me said to see her. So, I did.

My session made me curious and open to learning more about myself. So, I signed up for an upcoming retreat the counselor was leading in North Carolina.

The retreat started on a Friday afternoon. We got up at four on Saturday morning for an hour mediation session, yoga, and a light breakfast. Then, the leader said we were going on a hike, which cul-minated in our climbing a mountain.

The climb was challenging, but I was one of the first to make it to the top. As I sat in the tall, cool grass, I breathed in the fresh air and took in the extraordinary view.

Then it hit me . . .

The date was May 9—precisely one month from the day I had sat in the hospital parking lot and pled to be on top of a mountain.

I was in awe. The Universe had heard my emotional plea and found a way to respond to my desire. And for the first time in a long while, I cried tears of joy.

Sitting on top of that mountain was my high point (no pun in-tended) for the coming months. Losing my sister, who was also my confidant, left me feeling numb and out of sync. I stopped doing ac-tivities that reminded me of her—listening to seventies and eighties music, making our favorite childhood desserts, and dreaming about starting businesses.

For nearly a year, I did my best to avoid *anything* that would make me feel.

* * *

Eventually, I started to climb out of my grief. I was afraid of dying young like my sister, so I started a mission to lead a happier, health-ier, and more purposeful life.

My first steps involved changing my diet, meditating, and jour-naling. Slowly, I could feel myself reconnecting and enjoying life again.

Then, in early 2003, I took a bold step. I walked away from my eighteen-year career as an environmental scientist to become a free-lance copywriter.

When I told my friends, family, and boss about my decision, they were shocked. And I'm sure most of them were worried because, up until then, I had always made "smart" and "responsible" decisions.

No one knew I had never been passionate about my career. Sure, I was steadily climbing the corporate ladder, but I wasn't growing in the ways that were important to me. I yearned for freedom from the restrictions of corporate America. And I wanted to help people realize the power of their minds to enjoy bigger, bolder, and happier lives.

However, I knew that to enjoy true freedom, I would have to learn how to control my thoughts and expand my consciousness. My goal was to specialize in personal development to help me become the highest expression of myself while helping others.

My dream was to write for a company called Nightingale Conant, which had been around for nearly fifty years, producing audio programs for personal development leaders, including Tony Robbins, Wayne Dyer, and Jack Canfield. The company had changed the lives of millions worldwide. The thought of being involved with their work inspired me to change my career.

* * *

A year later, I attended a copywriting boot camp. While I was there, I met Dave, the president of a marketing company that helped new copywriters land projects. Dave asked me about my goals, and I mentioned that Nightingale Conant was my dream client.

Dave laughed and said, "They're ours, too! We've been trying to get a project with them for a couple of years. You're doing great work, so if we ever get a project with them, you'll be the first one I'll call."

Three weeks later, I experienced a magical moment.

Dave called to tell me his company had just landed their first assignment with Nightingale Conant. He said, "The project is yours if you want it."

For the first time since being on the mountaintop in 1999, I felt a solid connection to the Universe.

The first ten years of my copywriting career were everything I had hoped for—and more. The best part was becoming a go-to freelancer for Nightingale Conant for audio programs that dealt with spirituality, healing, and expanding consciousness. I loved the work so much that I often couldn't believe I was getting paid for it.

But then, the company took a hard hit during the 2008–2009 recession. And by late 2011, Nightingale no longer needed my help. It was a hard blow because not only was I losing the only "job" I had ever loved, but I also felt sad for the Nightingale employees who were losing *their* jobs.

Without Nightingale Conant in the picture, I didn't know what to do. I received offers for projects in lucrative industries (such as financial newsletters), but I turned them down.

I told myself I was saying "no" because I didn't know much about the industry. However, if I tell myself the truth, I didn't accept the projects because I was afraid I wouldn't do well, and my fear kept me from trying.

I didn't have any clear direction for my career for the next three years. I accepted whatever came along. Occasionally, I did freelance jobs for companies I was familiar with, and I also worked for an energy healer about twenty-four hours a week.

In early February of 2015, as I watched the Super Bowl, I had a flash of inspiration.

I knew what I wanted.

I ran upstairs and wrote in my journal: *I want to write full-time for a company like Nightingale Conant.*

To my surprise, three days later the Universe responded to my desire. The CEO of a major player in the personal development industry called me. She said a former copywriter for Nightingale had given her my name. The CEO asked if I wanted to become the company's copywriter.

I was excited to work for the company, so I took the job. I worked for the company as a full-time independent contractor for six years.

* * *

As I write this today, I've studied the teachings of more than a dozen well-known personal development experts on how to do *almost* everything a person needs to know and do to create the life of his or her dreams. And I've written "how to change your life" ideas that were shared with millions of people.

However, even though I knew how to write the words convincingly, I was not embodying the teachings. So my life was not a demonstration of what I had learned.

There's an idiom that says when you know better, you do better. But that's not necessarily true. There's often a gap between what we know and what we do. It's the gap between being stuck and getting free.

For years, I fell squarely in that gap. I knew (in my mind) what was possible, but I didn't act on it because I hadn't done the necessary work to bridge the knowing/doing gap—the emotional and mental work that would finally set me free.

Why?

Because I thought even if I allowed myself to fantasize about what I truly wanted in life, I wouldn't be good enough to reach my dreams. In my mind, not trying was better than failing. It was safer.

And so, I became a chameleon. I blended in with my environment and regurgitated the experts' words to help the people I was writing to transform *their* lives without internalizing those ideas to alter my own.

Now and then, I would play with the idea of starting my own

business, writing books, or coaching. But each time I got ready to do any of them, I began to squirm. I couldn't do it yet. I wasn't prepared.

2020

But life started to change on May 26—the day I heard about George Floyd's death. Watching the horrifying minutes that led to Mr. Floyd's last breaths and then witnessing people worldwide come together during a pandemic to protest the injustice was a wake-up call.

In the following days and weeks, something started to shift inside me. I was no longer willing to settle for where I was and what I was doing every day. I was determined to find a way to connect with myself again and feel more hopeful about the future.

* * *

I started my inner fitness journey in late June.

I read *The Little Book of Big Lies* and then started participating in Wellness Wednesday sessions. I noticed improvements in how I felt about and treated myself immediately. I took the next step and started doing Inner Fitness Workouts in July.

Finally, after all my years of working in personal development, the cloudy skies started to part and patches of sunlight began to shine brightly through. I had landed on something that connected with my soul.

Next, I signed up for an Inner Fitness Circle (IFC). The IFC members bonded immediately. The next day, we created a group text thread to motivate, support, and encourage one another to grow and engage in Self-care.

For the first few weeks of meeting with the IFC, I relied heavily on Practice 1—*I practice turning my life over to a power greater than me that loves me and responds to my heart.* This practice helped me see how cut off I was from my heart and feelings.

I used the remaining 13 practices to help me feel safe enough to get curious about what my heart wanted. Instead of running away from what my heart wanted to tell me, I started walking toward it in a loving and nonjudgmental way. I'm grateful that my heart trusts me again, and it openly speaks to me, letting me know how it feels and what it needs and wants.

The 14 Practices for Inner Health and Wellbeing provide practical tools to get to the truth behind decades of feeling disconnected, disappointed, and frustrated. And the IFC held me accountable for my growth—every week.

And now, for the first time in many years, I can latch onto new ideas and dreams that have the power to pull me forward.

When I started my inner fitness journey, I journaled more in six months than I did in the previous thirteen years. Doing this work is helping me find, develop, and use my voice.

I read a blog post recently that asked this question: *If we were to meet three years from now, what would have to happen in your life personally and professionally for you to be really happy about where you are?*

I wrote a page and a half in my journal in answer to that question. When I read what I wrote, I realized everything I had written could happen if I accomplished one thing . . . Self-mastery.

Then, I wrote in my journal:

Here's what I can do to become the master of myself:
- Pay attention to my thoughts, interrupt old patterns, and replace outdated ideas with perspectives that reveal new possibilities and create first-time experiences.
- Observe my life from an objective perspective and choose whether to keep things as they are or change them.

- Let go of petty thinking and small ideas, and commit to making the rest of my life my best years.
- Get curious about things that scare or challenge me.
- Decide what I want for my life, go for it, and have faith.

I never thought I'd say this, but I'm grateful for the enormous social and political challenges of 2020. The pain was so overwhelming that I knew that standing still was no longer an option if I was ever going to thrive. So, I started moving in a new direction that led to the Inner Fitness Project.

Now, I am paying attention to my thoughts, patterns, and feelings, and redirecting them when necessary to a more loving, accepting, and empowering perspective.

And the best part is I know my life will only get better from here as I continue to do my inner work and expand into higher expressions of myself.

Lisa: Silenced at Work

FROM DAY ONE, OR WHAT I REMEMBER DAY ONE TO BE, I have always been an extremely independent and outgoing person who made friends easily. I was comfortable with being honest with myself. Speaking my truth to others was a breeze. I quickly stood up for what was right and did not hesitate to speak out against what was wrong. I was taught to be confident, to believe in myself because I am to keep God first, and through God I can do all things. Believing this placed JOY in my heart. I carried this JOY every day of my life. As I grew older, this JOY showed up as a daily smile on my face and an approachable attitude. If not always, most often I felt joyous and happy, yet not for any particular reason. I was simply happy with myself.

As I grew older and began to live life, I soon realized that not everyone lived life through the same rose-tinted glasses. In college, a classmate once asked me, "Why do you always look so happy?" She stated that I was never upset or in a bad mood. I told her that statement wasn't true. At that point in life, I didn't really know how to explain the JOY that I felt, nor did I feel the need to defend or explain it. This young lady was still very confident that I was A-OK. The feelings and opinions of others did not matter much to me.

After college, I worked in a very male-dominated industry. Although my work was appreciated and I was paid well and recognized for my hard work, at times I did not feel seen and heard. Over time, this began to impact my JOY. It forced me to grow thick skin, yet to shrink a bit, depending on the situation.

Fast-forward to another job experience. This time the environment was different. In the beginning it was a breath of fresh air. I was managing a team. In that company, the leadership roles were filled with many women; there was an even playing field. Males and females equally held powerful positions. I thought, *AWESOME!* Hopeful for a great experience at that company, no longer feeling that I had to shrink myself, I felt that I was getting my level of JOY up! This type of energy carried on for a while, but as time went on, the unexpected happened. One day I found myself in an office with an HR specialist advising me to shrink myself to accommodate the insecurities of my manager. The words flowed from her lips with ease: "You tend to think faster than some people. Just because you know, you don't have to *say* that you know. You don't have to let everyone know that you know." I was floored. Yet again, I felt that I needed to shrink myself to get along in my career. It was crushing.

Through life I identified myself as a finance professional, daughter, sister, auntie, wife, mother, and friend. I took these titles seriously. I showed up accordingly. Eventually I realized that I showed up accordingly for everyone but myself. I had a list of things that I was passionate about, cared about deeply, and wanted for my future, but I continued to put them on the back burner. Most of them I did not think that I would ever have the bandwidth to get to. At the same time, I continued to show up for everyone else. This behavior continued for many years. Once COVID hit us all like a ton of bricks, I was able to spend more time with myself. I then realized that I was fed up with this feeling. I had put myself on the back burner for too long. I felt stuck.

During the COVID pandemic, I decided to join Instagram simply to watch Jill Scott and Erykah Badu perform. While browsing one day, I saw a familiar face—Tina Lifford. I noticed the Inner Fitness Project. This caught my attention, as I always had a huge interest in self-help books and resources. At that point in my life, after experiencing a few challenging people and events, I felt that I had lost some of the JOY in my heart. I felt stuck in a place where I continued to put myself last.

I decided to check out the Inner Fitness Project. I started by joining Wellness Wednesday sessions. These sessions were powerful, with great structure. After a few sessions, this felt like a safe, judgment-free space. The meeting is kicked off with greeting and centering. This is a time to let go of the stress of the day and relax a bit. A passage is read from a book, and attendees have the opportunity to speak about anything that resonates from the reading. After that, the floor is open for group sharing. This feels like a group therapy session. I felt I needed that. Shortly I learned that I could share and get helpful feedback from Tina, or I could listen to others share, listen to Tina give feedback to others, and still receive what I've heard as a learning opportunity. This taught me that our experiences are similar and connected. I no longer felt alone or much different from others, with my list of challenges and roadblocks that I face. It became apparent that we are all humans, facing human experiences while responding with the human brain. Life is constantly bumping into life for all of us. It is how we choose to respond that makes the difference.

I acknowledged that I was making good progress with focusing on myself more through Wellness Wednesdays. The fact that I consistently built the habit of carving time out for myself every Wednesday at 9:00 p.m. was a huge WIN for me. I had to pat myself on the back for doing that. Within this time, I learned to use

"I" language, which helped me to feel accountable for my feelings. I was also reassured that I did not need to prove anything to anyone but simply share what I know to build community. For me, these were game-changers in the way that I started to show up. As a result of Wellness Wednesdays, I successfully built a new healthy habit. I was showing up for myself! This was significant.

After some time of consistently attending Wellness Wednesdays, I began to feel less stuck. I decided to apply to be a part of an Inner Fitness Circle and was eventually placed in a Circle full of amazing women. We were given guidelines, which included 14 Practices that were thoughtfully crafted to teach us how to show up more fully alive in everyday life. The guidelines ensured that each participant felt safe, seen, and heard in the space. We met weekly for about three months. Each week, I was able to choose one of the 14 Practices that I felt would help me work through where I was that week with any issues, challenges, or roadblocks. I found Practice 3 most helpful—*I embrace the idea that I am more than any challenge I face*. This experience had a powerful impact on my life. Not only did I begin to feel unstuck, but I was able to build new habits that put me on a path that led me back to being myself with songs of JOY in my heart. Along with all this, I built a lasting and divinely assembled bond with the women in this Circle.

Being a part of the Inner Fitness Project has done so much in my life. I've found the JOY that I lost many years ago. I am no longer defined and consumed by any of the hats I wear or titles I go by. I am Lisa. My focus is to show up as my authentic Self as life bumps into life, while not caring about the feelings and opinions of others.

I am grateful for Tina Lifford and the 14 Practices, as well as the community of the Inner Fitness Project. This platform has forever changed me for the better. I can see the impact by the way that I show up for myself and for others. A bonus is that these differences in me have spilled over and positively influenced my loved ones. My household is forever changed. For example, the communication between my husband and me is much more effective. We listen to understand, rather than choosing to listen to respond. This is exciting work. I look forward to expanding into my greater yet-to-be with the tools and practices of the Inner Fitness Project.

Renee: My Mother's Betrayal

I T WAS A TYPICAL SUMMER DAY IN THE LATE 1970S, ETCHED in my memory, which unfolded with the clarity that only moments of profound change possess. I was at the sink, hands submerged in soapy water, lost in washing dishes. My outfit—a pair of brown windowpane bell-bottom jeans and a tie-dyed back-out top, a gift from my mother—felt like a second skin, a vibrant testament to the era's fashion and my youthful innocence.

The air was thick with heat, a typical feature of those long summer afternoons in LA. I was eleven years old, and my body was on the cusp of womanhood, caught in the awkward stage of early development, a fact I was only dimly aware of and hardly ready to navigate.

The house was filled with the usual sounds: the distant hum of traffic outside, the low murmur of the radio playing the Bee Gees' "How Deep Is Your Love," a melody I found myself singing along to in perfect harmony, lost in the music and the simplicity of the moment. My mother's new boyfriend was seated at our formal dining room table. My mother was in the bathroom, preparing for their date, her voice occasionally drifting out to where he sat, a lifeline between them that somehow excluded me.

From my vantage point in the kitchen, invisible to my mother yet fully visible to her boyfriend, I was oblivious to the unfolding drama, ensconced in my own world. Then, without warning, my mother burst into the kitchen, her hand striking my face with a force that sent me tumbling to the ground. The shock of the cold floor against my skin was nothing compared to the confusion and terror that gripped me as I looked up into her face—a face I barely recognized, twisted into an expression of anger and accusation.

She accused me of flaunting myself before her boyfriend, interpreting his gaze as evidence of my guilt. The absurdity of the accusation left me reeling. How could she believe such a thing? How could the simple act of standing in my kitchen in clothes she had chosen for me twist into something so vile?

In that moment of betrayal and pain, my first thought was to tell my mother, and that is when a fundamental truth shattered within me: I was no longer safe in my own home. The realization that my mother, the one person in the world who was supposed to protect and cherish me, was now the source of my most profound hurt was a wound far deeper than the physical sting of her slap.

The innocence of my childhood crumbled away under the weight of her unfounded accusations. The realization that I was alone, truly alone, in navigating the complexities of growing up was a heavy burden on an eleven-year-old's shoulders. The person who had nourished me, loved me, and cared for me was now the person causing me pain. In the aftermath of her slap, the remnants of my trust and security lay scattered around me like broken glass, marking the end of my childhood and the beginning of a journey through a world that had suddenly become much more complicated and unforgiving.

After that slap, my room became my refuge, not by choice but by necessity. It was a sanctuary imposed upon me as I was relegated to its confines whenever her boyfriends visited—unlike my brothers, who were too young to recognize what was happening and were free to exist as they always had.

Isolated, I often found myself pressing an ear against the cold wall, straining to catch snippets of my mother's conversations. Often, she was on the phone with someone. Those conversations became my window into how she truly viewed me. The words she spoke about me were like daggers, each sentence another slice into the fabric of my soul. She painted an unrecognizable picture of me, attributing actions and attitudes to me that were as foreign as they were hurtful.

The ritual humiliation didn't end with verbal slander; physical abuse followed, often while I was in the bathtub, when she would burst through the door. The instruments of my punishment varied—a Hot Wheels track or a belt—but the intention behind them was always the same: to inflict pain and fear. Naked and defenseless, I endured those beatings, a stark and painful contrast to the sanctity that bath time is supposed to represent for a child.

And yet, every Sunday morning, we would don our best clothes and head to church as if nothing had ever happened. I would stand in front of the congregation, singing lead in the choir. My voice, clear and strong, belied the turmoil that churned within me, a testament to the duality of my existence.

I have had moments when I contemplated suicide. Once, when I was seventeen, I lived in my own apartment and worked two low-paying fast-food jobs. Living in a high crime area had its challenges, such as having to stand at bus stops at all hours because I didn't have a car. Still, it was better than sleeping in my friends' garages at night and leaving before their parents opened the garage to retrieve their cars for work in the morning, or sleeping in my mom's backyard on the patio swing with a blanket that I kept hidden in the tool shed nearby.

There was no refuge from the pain I was still feeling internally, so one night, overwhelmed by exhaustion and fear, I found myself feeling nothing but isolation and despair. It seemed as though life had dealt me a bad hand, leaving me questioning why I had to endure such hardships. In a moment of desperation, I attempted to end my suffering by consuming a mixture of pills, including painkillers. As I began to lose consciousness, doubts flooded my mind. I was haunted by the belief that suicide was a sin that would condemn me to eternal torment. Fearing this outcome, I reached out to my cousin, who lived nearby. This led to a three-day stay in the hospital, and after that, neither my parents nor I ever brought it up.

As 2020 ended, I found myself in the suburbs of Atlanta, living what I had once envisioned as my dream life. My home, with its five bedrooms, three and a half baths, theater room, sunroom, screened porch, and stunning pool, was designed to be the envy of all who knew me. Yet, I encountered the familiar foes of isolation and despair within these walls. The grandeur of my surroundings did little to quell the turmoil within; if anything, it magnified my sense of loneliness. The thought of enduring another moment of such anguish was unbearable. Unlike before, the fear of eternal torment no longer held sway over me; my life itself felt like an unending trial.

The depths of my sorrow hadn't been plumbed since the loss of my mother in 2017, a testament to the profound impact of cumulative grief and unresolved trauma. Despite the external changes in my life, the internal patterns remained unbroken, leading me to contemplate a final escape from the pain. The realization that I had never stayed in one place for more than three years struck me, highlighting a cycle of flight without respite. Exhaustion had set in, sapping the strength needed to start anew and pushing me to the brink.

In that moment of despair, I considered the possibility that I was the problem, perhaps as flawed and unstable as some had suggested throughout my life. Therapy alone was not working. So what else was left? Then, I recalled a book by Tina Lifford that spoke to the multifaceted nature of the Self: the surviving self, the thriving Self, and the infinite SELF. Lifford's words had struck a chord, resonating with my own fragmented experience.

Driven by a mix of desperation and hope, I sought out Lifford's Inner Fitness Project on Instagram. Joining that community represented my final attempt at salvaging my will to live. It was my last try at life, and I knew it. And much to my surprise, that decision marked the beginning of a transformative journey. The project offered more than just coaching; it was a collective endeavor involving women from diverse backgrounds, all united by their struggles. Despite differences in education and life paths, our shared experiences of pain and search for peace bridged any gaps between us.

This sense of connection was revelatory. Hearing the stories of others, women who were educated, successful, and outwardly composed yet shared my feelings of inadequacy and turmoil, I began to see my own experiences in a new light. The realization dawned on me that my feelings of being an outsider, of being "crazy," were unfounded. My reactions and emotions were normal responses to the extraordinary challenges I had faced.

The Inner Fitness Project became a beacon of hope, a place where the act of sharing and listening fostered a sense of belonging and understanding. It taught me that healing isn't a solitary journey but a communal one, where the strength of others can bolster my own. This community, this mental gym, equipped me with the tools to confront my past, understand my present, and envision a future where peace isn't just a fleeting dream but a tangible reality. For the first time in a long while, I felt normal, validated, and, most important, hopeful.

Embarking on this journey with the Inner Fitness Project was far from easy. Tina Lifford challenged us with questions that forced me to confront truths I would have ignored. It wasn't a straightforward path; numerous pivotal moments tested my resolve. Despite periods of feeling uplifted, I frequently found myself spiraling back into the depths of depression, anxiety, and panic attacks. A particularly raw moment came when I broke down in front of the group, confessing my fear that despite my best efforts, nothing seemed to be changing.

Tina's response to my despair was a turning point. She explained that the damaging beliefs and lies I had internalized over the years had deeply rooted themselves in my subconscious, playing cruel tricks on my perception of reality. Her guidance during our sessions began to pierce through these layers of deception, offering glimpses of clarity and understanding.

One session stands out vividly in my memory. My words, though now forgotten, prompted Tina to address me with a mix of sternness and profound love—like that of a grandmother, mother, sister, and friend all rolled into one. Her emotional plea for me to stop beating myself up was a powerful moment. She likened my self-criticism to the whippings inflicted by slave owners, urging me to cease treating myself with such cruelty. Her words struck a chord, marking the first time I truly grasped that I held the power to change how I treated myself, regardless of past experiences.

Another breakthrough occurred during an exercise where Tina asked us to write down our responses to a particular question. Though I can't recall what I wrote, the act of writing unleashed a torrent of tears and a profound realization: *I didn't like myself.* This insight forced me to confront the uncomfortable truth that I had been seeking love and validation from others without first learning to love myself. My subconscious mind had been concealing this reality, perpetuating an internal conflict that I was now determined to resolve.

Understanding that the surviving self—the part of me that had endured so much—was not my enemy but a protector who loved me deeply was liberating. It was a crucial step toward internal harmony, allowing space for all parts of me to coexist peacefully.

To reinforce this newfound understanding and integrate it into my daily life, I turned to Tina's 14 Practices. I wrote them on sticky notes and plastered them all over my bathroom mirror and home office. These reminders served as daily workouts of my commitment to healing, to treating myself with kindness, and to fostering a love for myself that had been absent for decades. These practices weren't just about self-improvement; they were a declaration of self-love and a vow to break the cycle of internalized negativity.

Practice 7—*I release all people and things from the responsibility of making me happy*—became a pivotal mantra in my journey of self-discovery and healing. I would find myself spiraling down a dark hole because someone left me or I felt betrayed by a loved one, and I would just lie down in a fetal position feeling powerless; but this practice empowered me to take ownership of my happiness and accomplishments, freeing me from the weight of external expectations and past disappointments. This mindset shift enabled me to revisit and achieve goals that had been dormant for years, marking significant milestones in my personal growth.

As I navigated this process, the changes in how I perceived myself and interacted with the world were profound. I was building a foundation not just for survival but for a life filled with purpose and joy. This transformation also paved the way for forgiveness and understanding toward my mother. Recognizing that she, too, was a victim of early trauma, I began to see her actions and limitations through a lens of compassion. When I understood the impact of unresolved trauma and considered my own decades-long journey to enlightenment, empathy for her struggle came naturally to me. It became clear that she had loved me in the best way she knew, given her circumstances.

Incorporating Practice 14—*I cultivate social connections where I feel safe, seen, and heard*—into my life was another crucial step. I learned how vital it was for me to set boundaries. This practice helped me establish a supportive network that provided me with a sense of belonging, and for the first time, I experienced what it truly meant to be at peace with myself and my past. Realizing that I could rely on my inner strength and resilience was liberating. Knowing that "as long as I got me, I'm okay" instilled a profound sense of self-assurance and prepared me to pursue my dreams.

Reflecting on my journey, I feel a deep sense of pride in the person I've become. The decision to pick up Tina Lifford's book and commit to the challenging yet rewarding process of the Inner Fitness Project was a defining moment in my life. It wasn't just about healing; it was about discovering myself, learning to love and forgive, and ultimately, finding peace. Now, I have more good days than bad ones, and when I do find myself feeling low and can't seem to pick myself up, I just let it pass through me. I refuse to let it define me. I am proud of Renee, who embarked on this path a few years ago, who persevered through the highs and lows and emerged stronger and more self-aware. This journey has not only transformed my relationship with myself but has also opened the door to a future where I can thrive and finally live out my dreams. It's always possible to change. I'm gonna be alright!

Ruth: Becoming Well

I AM A FIFTY-SIX-YEAR-OLD BUTCH LESBIAN; I HAVE BEEN clean and sober for thirty-one years. I am blessed to have three children and nine grandchildren. I am the oldest child of deaf parents; I have two sisters and one half-brother; and I'm currently in the midst of supporting my mother through her terminal congestive heart failure and transition.

Thirty-six years ago, I never would have imagined my life to be what it is today. I am forever grateful for my sobriety and the gift of many lessons throughout the years. The gift of these lessons continues to remind me of how precious life is and the beauty of being fully present in the pain, joy, and glory of living my most authentic life. It has not always been easy. Until about five years ago, I felt the need to scratch and fight my way to be seen, heard, and loved.

When I was eight or nine years old, my father's best friend started sexually molesting me. Not too long after that, the neighborhood men began sexually abusing my sisters and me, in addition to our pediatrician. I was afraid to tell my mom and dad about the sexual abuse because my father's best friend threatened to kill my sisters and both my parents if I did. I lived with these painful secrets for many years until I sought therapy when I was eighteen.

In my early sessions with my first therapist, Linda, I was so traumatized by my childhood abuse that I could not sit alone in a room with her and talk about it. I needed our sessions to be outdoors in an open space, so I had the room to breathe through it. If we were in a closed room, I had to sit by the door, and I asked that she sit in the chair farthest from the door. I always needed a way to escape if the work became too painful or too difficult. She is an amazing human, and we worked together on and off for many years.

When I was nineteen years old, I got pregnant and chose to give my daughter up for adoption. This was the most painful and excruciating choice I've ever made, but it was the best choice for my daughter. I was struggling with my addictions, surviving, and reacting to my childhood traumas and their painful results. I was in no position to be raising and parenting another human being. I had decided to move forward with an open adoption, and at the time, that was unheard-of, but I would not settle for anything less.

I had been carrying the weight of my family's generational abuse, traumas, and hurt my whole life, and I did not want my daughter to know that pain, in the same way I had come to know my family's pain. I gave my child up to spare her soul and break our generational curse of verbal and physical abuse. I was determined to protect my child's emotional and mental stability at any cost; however, I was not prepared for the loss and heartbreaking grief that followed. I continued to work with my therapist; she helped me stay grounded in the truth and purpose of why I gave her up for adoption. Linda helped me rewire my pain from grief to gratitude.

As the oldest child growing up in a family with deaf parents, I was required to be present and interpret for my parents at a moment's notice. From an early age, I was often pulled out of school to help my parents communicate when paying the utilities. I was also required to interpret for all doctor visits for my sisters and my parents, as well as any other appointments where they needed me to communicate for them. Most of my extended family members had always relied on us kids to communicate their arguments, dysfunction, and basic dialogue rather than taking the responsibility of learning sign language so they could communicate with my parents directly.

As a result of this imposed and unwanted family role, my educational needs and other areas of my life were not recognized or honored. I resented being the oldest child, and I resented all of the responsibilities this role required. I hated interpreting for my parents. As I grew older, my role morphed into an all-encompassing responsibility to parent my deaf parents.

In my experience, growing up with deaf parents created many cultural and emotional expectations that are unreasonable and, in some ways, psychologically and emotionally abusive. I was exposed to situations that no child should be exposed to; I was expected to care for my siblings on a level that was beyond my capabilities; and I was denied my basic right to just be a child and to focus on my education.

I've struggled in school my whole life. Early on, stigmatism in my eyes prevented me from seeing what was on the chalkboard, causing me to misinterpret lessons and later come up with incorrect answers. My teachers often ridiculed and criticized me, until they discovered that I needed glasses, but my academic struggles did not end there.

I am a deeply sensitive human, both physically and emotionally. As a child, I had no idea that I was an empath or how to manage it. At the age of twelve, I was deeply traumatized by our move from Kentucky to California. When I spoke, I had a heavy Southern drawl, and that was a great source of pain when I entered seventh grade in Southern California.

My naïve hillbilly psyche was no match for the cruel and unkind OP (Ocean Pacific) shorts-wearing, cool, California surfer and skateboarder type of kids I went to school with. They were relentless in their cruelty and bullying behavior. They often made fun of me for the way that I spoke and how I looked and dressed. This was true culture shock. The fact that I was always struggling with my classes and getting bad grades did not support a healthy and loving self-esteem.

In addition to the educational culture shock, we were forced to move into my maternal grandmother's home (we called her Maw-Maw). In my short life of twelve years, I had never been exposed to such toxic and cruel verbal abuse. MawMaw was the most unhappy and unkind person I have ever known, still to this day. She was the most racist, homophobic, woman-hating, man-hating, [fill in the blank]-hating and hateful person one could ever know. She would pit her children and grandchildren against one another, and she would take great joy in the divisive and cruel games she played with her family. MawMaw would make fun of my deaf parents with us in the room; she hated my mother for being deaf and resented the relationship my mom and I had with her sister, my great-aunt Ruth (whom I called Grandma Ruth).

In addition to living with MawMaw, we lived with Uncle Herb, who lived with MawMaw and was an alcoholic. We were constantly exposed to his combative and abusive relationship with MawMaw and, of course, anyone else who crossed him during one of his drunken tirades. Without fail, when my uncle received his disability check at the first of the month, MawMaw would make us kids go looking for him every night to pull him out of local bars and bring him home. Sometimes we didn't have to go far because we would find him face down in the middle of the street or in the gutter, mumbling expletives. Then we would help carry him home, often bloody and battered from a barroom brawl or fall.

I barely passed or failed most of my classes in ninth grade, with the exception to geography. I loved geography, I loved to travel, and I loved reading maps. I was labeled as a troubled student and for my tenth-grade year was sent to the school where all the other troubled kids went. When I failed tenth grade, I went on to take correspondence classes (a.k.a. homeschooling) in the eleventh grade. I quit school during the eleventh grade.

It wasn't until much later in life that I discovered I had a learning disability—a form of dyslexia. I was never officially diagnosed, but it was a life-changing moment when I realized that I was not as stupid as everyone thought, including myself. I was always in survival mode and did not have the capacity or know-how to ask for help. In the early 1990s I was introduced to Microsoft Word and its spell-checker. That was another great moment in my life—as a matter of fact, it was life-changing. The first letter I ever wrote on a computer was riddled with misspellings and red lines from top to bottom. Thank GOD for spell-check! It was the first time I saw in print what everyone else saw; everything started to make sense.

Grandma Ruth is my greatest hero, and I am her namesake. I call her "grandma" because she was the closest person to me, the person who raised my mother, and the person I spent my childhood with. Grandma Ruth was my protector; she protected me from many things, and I experienced nothing but unconditional love and adoration from her. As a child, I traveled extensively with my grandparents Ruth and Elliott; they are the sole reason that my love of travel and adventure was birthed. When my parents moved us from the Midwest to California, they removed me from the only loving and protective environment I had ever known.

My therapist Linda saved my life many times over. She loved me through my initial healing and survival work, she helped me through my pregnancy when my entire family abandoned me, and she gave me the basic tools I needed to seek and maintain my sobriety. Linda supported and encouraged me to go back to school and get my GED; I am forever grateful for Linda's patience, love, and kindness.

Many years later, and well into my healing journey, I was finally ready for children. While living in Chicago, I became a foster parent, and at the age of thirty-five, I adopted two biological brothers. These two beautiful souls changed my life. It was not easy being a single parent and raising two boys with a troubled past. Our journey has had many challenges, but I love them with every ounce of my heart and soul. I am so grateful for both of them, and the honor and gift it has been to be their mother.

About five years ago, I was unexpectedly catapulted onto a healing path that was brought on by a deep betrayal of friends and an industry giant in my moto community. As a result, I was introduced to my current life coach, Cynthia James. Working with Cynthia James has been healing and transformative on so many levels, and I'm forever grateful for her love and support, and the work we've accomplished together. But despite positive changes, patterns of betrayal kept showing up in my workplace and relationships, over and over again.

About two and a half years ago, I experienced a layoff with the company that I'd been with for almost ten years. But then an opportunity came up for me to relocate and work with the same company in Mississippi. I jumped at this opportunity because I needed a job, and I wanted to continue working with my company. This was a difficult transition, as I had to leave my family and the only community I had known for more than thirty years. I was also working on a film project that I had stepped into without any experience, just a heart full of desire, courage, and great intentions.

Unfortunately, through a series of events beyond my control, I slipped into a deep depression and shame spiral. I allowed my film project to suffer, and I continued to mistreat myself through harsh, self-deprecating language, using food as my "spiritual guide," and residing in a functionally depressing existence. After two years in Mississippi, I experienced more personal betrayal and another lay-off. Please, not again!

Last year, at the Women Creating Our Futures conference, Cynthia James introduced me to her dear friend of thirty years and amazing life coach Tina Lifford. I learned about Tina's book *The Little Book of Big Lies* and signed up for her newsletter. About a year later, I was still in the midst of my depression; when I saw an email about an Inner Fitness Workout called "Interrupting Old Patterns," I signed up right away. Through this workout, I recognized my need to shift and refocus my energy. I needed to reengage and create a different strategy for the next phase of my life. I love the simplicity of the workouts and the depth of the work and message. So I signed up for a series of ten Inner Fitness Workouts.

While signing up for this series, I also saw an invitation to be-come part of an Inner Fitness Circle beta program and was excited to learn more about it. I had chosen many different paths through the years to help keep me clean and sober, but I wish that the Inner Fitness Circle had been available to me twenty-five-plus years ago.

Once I started the Inner Fitness Circle meetings, I felt emo-tionally safe, seen, and encouraged in a completely nonjudgmental environment. This was different from the other kinds of meetings I had been a part of throughout my healing. Each week during the three months of Circle meetings, I chose one of the 14 Practices to focus on to remind me of my worth.

In one lesson, I had been dating a woman for several months who I believed had been lying and emotionally cheating on me. During one of our Inner Fitness Workouts, I was able to identify my knee-jerk reactions and how I hadn't been honoring or listening to my intuitive Self, which was telling me to stop dating this woman. She wasn't meeting my needs, and her aloofness and dismissive communication habits triggered me.

I came to see how I wasn't honoring my own needs, listening to my intuition, trusting, loving, and supporting my desire for a partner who would care about what I needed for connection and communication. Shifting my focus away from another person and going inward was critical to me for making that transition. I came to see how my triggers controlled the outcome, my reactions fed the fury, and my fear of heartbreak (yet one more time) crippled my judgment and execution of Self-love.

I stayed in self-doubt, and I spent a lot of time on Practice 10—*I become a great parent and friend to myself.* In this work, I was able to see and honor my intuition and needs. Later, I also applied Practice 8—*I ask to profoundly accept my Self and believe in my value*—which helped me be able to give myself permission to let go of old patterns and the habit of hanging on to the lie that I was not worthy of someone treating me with love, kindness, and respect. I released that woman and honored *me.*

I am so grateful for this amazing platform, the 14 Practices, and the Inner Fitness Workouts. I now know that I do not have to live in the Big Lies I've been telling myself.

Stay tuned—I am in the process of becoming a masterpiece!

Sharon: Depression

I TURNED FIFTY IN THE SUMMER OF 2020. I HAD BEEN LOOK-ing forward to that milestone birthday for years. I envisioned myself celebrating with friends, taking a big vacation, and welcoming this new season with excitement. Instead, my birthday came four months after the coronavirus was declared a pandemic. I was locked in an oppressively hot house with a broken air conditioner in the middle of the summer, literally fearing for my life and the lives of everyone else. I was bombarded with stories of death, illness, and societal chaos. I spent my birthday on Zoom with a few family members and friends, trying to smile and pretend that I was okay, even though I was sad and terrified.

Over the next few years, the world eventually moved into a "new normal," and people seemed determined to live their best lives and put the pandemic behind them. But not only was I not successfully moving into the "new normal," I was also falling deeper into a depression. I stayed locked in my house for two years, working from home, isolated, and seeing no one except my husband. By the beginning of 2023, I was completely burned out. I could not focus or concentrate. I had insomnia. I quit three different jobs in the span of three years, which is significant because I usually stay with a job for at least ten years. To top it all off, I was going through physical and hormonal changes due to the onset of menopause. I was regularly envisioning myself getting in my car, driving far away to an unknown destination, and never coming back.

When I quit my job at the beginning of 2023, I decided to take a real break and focus on getting myself healthy. To be transparent, I did not actually "decide" to take a break. Saying it in that way makes it sound rational. In fact, I felt like I crashed into a wall, fell to the ground, and was lying there watching the room spin. I felt defeated, weak, unstable, and embarrassed. Embarrassed because everything that I was feeling and experiencing was the opposite of what anyone who knows me would ever expect. To friends and family, I was the strong, rational, responsible, stable, calm person who had it all together. I could manage anything and do it with a smile. How could this happen to me?

I thought it was one of the worst years of my life. I felt guilty about quitting my job and taking a significant and unprecedented eight-month break from working. For the first several months, my thoughts were racing and unrelenting. *What's wrong with you? You're fifty-three years old. You can't just quit your job. Why can't you get it together? Why can't you pull yourself out of this depression? You were always so strong and now you're being weak and irresponsible. And what's so terrible about your life anyway? You must be going crazy. You should be ashamed of yourself!* I would not spend time with anyone who talked to me that way, and yet I talked to myself that way every single day.

I had to admit to myself that the pandemic did not create any of my issues and that's why the end of the pandemic did not make them go away. The pandemic brought to the surface the issues that had been brewing inside of me for many years. I had been working long hours in stressful jobs that I did not enjoy. I continued to go to school at the same time, getting one degree after another, pushing myself harder and harder. I worked hard to please my husband and make him happy. I spent hours on the phone listening to other people complain, rant, and rave about their lives. I spent little time with family and friends, and almost no time doing the things that I enjoyed or taking care of myself. I was completely out of balance, and I knew that I needed help.

If there had not been a pandemic, I would not have found my way to the Inner Fitness Project community. During the lockdown of 2020, I was desperately searching for positive and inspirational news and information online. I am not on social media, so I must be intentional and creative when I am looking for information. I began virtually attending a weekly online webinar that Iyanla Vanzant and Tina Lifford were co-hosting called "Love from a Distance." Consequently, I ended up on a distribution email list, and for years, I received emails advertising programs from the inner fitness community. It was not until the beginning of 2023, the same week that I quit my job to take an official mental health break, when I decided to sign up for Inner Fitness 101. Afterward, I read *The Little Book of Big Lies* by Tina Lifford, and I joined the SELF365 Inner Fitness program.

I started the SELF365 program feeling anxious, insecure, and confused. I was uncomfortable and nervous to speak to a group of strangers about my pain and personal struggles. I was doubtful that the program could help me because the format and guidelines were very different from anything that I had ever experienced. I understood therapy and counseling, but this was not either. I understood Christian-based groups that focused on biblical principles and prayer, but this program was not that either. It was an opportunity for me to be in a small group with people who were quite different from one another, and yet were all experiencing similar issues. Being in a group of people who were willing to be so open and honest about their pain and life experiences was new and refreshing. It is exceedingly rare, even among family and close friends, for people to be truly honest about what is going on with them. Together, we learned and practiced new ways of thinking and processing our lives in a kind, supportive environment.

By the end of the fourteen-week SELF365 program, I had many specific tools and practices that I use every day to change my self-critical way of thinking and perceiving life. I developed an awareness and acceptance of myself, and I no longer talk to myself in ways that are harsh, unloving, and counterproductive. When I first started the program, I felt guilty for taking the time to focus on myself. I thought it was vain and selfish. I now understand that focusing on my mental and emotional health is not selfish. Yet, when I found out about the inner fitness weekend retreat that was happening at the end of the summer of 2023, my first instinct was to talk myself out of going. I thought, *I cannot afford that now. I'm not working. I won't know most of the people there. I won't fit in. And it isn't a good idea for me to drive seven hours by myself into the mountains of North Carolina.*

My husband had been watching my stress and struggles for years and witnessed the positive impact that the Inner Fitness Project was having in my life, so he offered to drive me to the retreat and help me pay for it. I decided to go. Working on various exercises all weekend with the women at the retreat was emotionally draining for me and difficult. Yet, it was exactly what I needed. The exercises seemed so simple on the surface, but they were profound. It was a powerful, positive learning experience for me. Putting forth that effort showed me that I was valuable and worth the investment.

Taking time off and starting this journey gave me the best present I could ever receive—space. I stopped racing, running, achieving, accomplishing, worrying, analyzing, and planning. I stopped filling up my calendar to the point that I couldn't think straight. I got still and silent for months, and it was scary, weird, and wonderful. The stillness, silence, and space that I created for myself changed my life. I will never be perfect, and my life will never be free from adversity and pain. However, I'm fully equipped to handle anything that comes my way.

Two months ago, my father passed away. The months leading up to his passing were some of the most difficult months of my life. In fact, the weeks right before his death were the saddest days of my life. We had an estranged relationship, and I was shocked at the excruciating pain that I felt witnessing the end of his life. However, I was equally shocked that God showed up in such a powerful way and carried me through that experience. The space that I had created and the acceptance I had developed made me open and available to hear from God and accept his guidance. It enabled me to find peace and healing afterward. Storms will most definitely continue to come, but without the storms, I cannot grow.

The practices that I have learned and the growth that I have experienced are priceless to me. I am not where I want to be, but I have come a mighty long way. I am grateful to Tina Lifford and the Inner Fitness Project for encouraging me to start becoming the best version of me that I can be. I am looking forward to the rest of my journey with hope, faith, acceptance, peace, and a greater trust in myself and God.

Stephanie: My Mate's Death

———

IT WAS JUNE 16, 2020, THREE MONTHS AFTER BEING FORCED into COVID lockdown, when staying home those extra-long hours started messing with my state of mind.

I realized I needed to use this time to find a lifeline to bring me back to a place of joy and happiness. I desperately needed something to help change the thought cycle of negativity, uncertainty, and hopelessness.

Yes, I believe in God, but I also believe the higher power is bigger than what religion had previously fed me, and I needed more. So I started thinking about my previous years at Agape Spiritual Center during my marriage and realized I really missed everything about it, especially being surrounded by what I like to call progressive spiritual thinkers. I logged onto Instagram to send Michael Beckwith a short message and saw his post Lifting the Veil. In the video, he was conversing with a woman whom I've come to know as Tina Lifford.

Listening to their conversation about inner Self-care immediately awakened my spirit. Tina's words about valuing Self, with a capital S, were a missing note in my song. However, it was her profound statement "When you realize that attacking yourself is literally a rejection of God" that grabbed my attention down to the seat of my soul. Their discussion was on such a higher spiritual level, and it struck a chord with my inner being. Somehow, I translated the conversation to mean: "How you show up in life shows how much you love God." This is when I made the affirmative decision to learn more about what Ms. Lifford was sharing. And this led me to the truth inside *The Little Book of Big Lies*.

* * *

Growing up there was no way I would have thought that during my life I would endure what I've finally come to admit was trauma. This was my pity party, and I believed I had every right to feel like the victim.

My first trauma took place in the seventies during summer break at the age of fourteen. I witnessed my older brother, seventeen, get stabbed to death in a street brawl. The vision of him being stabbed in the throat, staggering, and falling to the sidewalk in a pool of blood is a nightmare that I have never been able to erase. This first experience with death included my having to testify at the court trial, which ended in what I now realize was an unjust verdict.

The animal that killed my brother was convicted of second-degree murder and only spent a short time behind bars. My family tried to make life as normal as possible, though I could see the pain clearly in my parents' eyes. There was never a conversation that took place to help heal our souls.

Life continued plunging ahead even though I felt like I wore a scarlet letter all through high school, where I was recognized as the girl whose brother had been killed.

* * *

In 2005, I married an amazing man. It seemed as if a force had assigned him to help shift my spiritual thinking and make me aware of a higher consciousness. There were days I reluctantly resisted and struggled with insecurities. Somehow, I also found dysfunctional comfort in just being stuck in the fears that religion had embedded in my thinking.

Ten years later, I hit rock bottom with the loss of my husband. My marriage was taken away by the devastating disease of cancer. I was not prepared to face what the next chapters of my life held for me. There was no plan, life insurance, or concrete employment or career, but somehow, I managed to survive day after day. I also had no idea I would feel so much torment. This affliction turned to depression, which led to my joining a grief support group at a local church. The support I received was helpful and carried me so that I could keep functioning enough to work and return home to bury myself in the obstructive pleasures of hopelessness, disinterest, overeating, anxiety, fatigue, and basking in thoughts of the end.

One year later, I decided to tackle all the unfinished benchmarks in my life and returned to school, which distracted me from my depression. Learning became the beginning of a new lifeline. Through my studies, I gained a deeper understanding of my husband's strength and intellectual greatness. Basically, I was finally able to understand the reason for our connection and how he was used in so many ways to try to help me expand, though I failed miserably. I succeeded in my studies, but I still felt grief had a strong grip on me. Every day, I managed but struggled to do simple daily activities. I didn't care about my appearance or what other folks thought or were doing.

* * *

In 2020, I was still functioning like a zombie, doing the same ole thing on a different day, internally at my wit's end, unhappy, and emotionally disconnected from life. I was missing my best friend and biggest supporter. I didn't know how to live life without him. This drove me to the journey of finding Self. I needed to learn how to fill the hole in my heart and feel a transformational change.

Immediately after watching the Instagram interview, I went online and signed up to attend my first Wellness Wednesday on June 17, 2020. I couldn't believe this opportunity came my way, and I accepted it as a universal sign. As I logged into the Zoom session, it immediately felt like I landed at the right place. I listened to Tina speak from a place of concern for each and every person who dared to enter the room. She spoke life to everyone, from her heart and soul, with words of wisdom and inspiration. The language connected and reinforced my decision to trust the process and the greater force that guided me toward inner fitness. That evening I was hooked and knew God had directed me to take this journey.

I showed up for Wellness Wednesday weekly, no matter how tired, depressed, or lazy I felt. I forced myself to show up for myself because I could feel the shift inside. Sometimes, I asked questions, and some days, I just listened and learned from others' situations. Tina's guidance was not just words; she created transformation tools designed to change negative and abusive thinking, and shift beyond your surviving self.

As the months flowed by, I continued to log into the Wellness Wednesday meetings, feeling stronger and more optimistic about life. Looking back, I can see that I was actually ready to receive the healing that Tina provided. It had shown up after my morning cries asking for help. Following Practice 11—*I tell myself the truth about what happened, my interpretation, how I feel, and what's possible*—

takes courage. Removing the mask meant telling the truth and not hiding behind lies, pretentiousness, and inauthenticity. What I had labeled failures in my life were all part of the lie. Don't get me wrong, it wasn't always easy to look at myself and tell the truth, but I did, and this carried me to the next stages of recovering.

Each week, I followed Tina's advice, practices, and guidelines. I kept a journal; wrote down my dreams, desires, and expectations; and learned how to choose to respond to circumstances in different ways that were supportive of me. Let me start by telling you it required putting in the work and the desire to want to change. The discipline to be accountable to me first made it possible to show up for others.

* * *

The hardest practice to grasp was Practice 10—*I become a great parent and friend to myself.* I couldn't wrap my head around this practice and didn't understand how to do the work to be that good friend. I always considered myself to be a great friend to those who were in my life. After all, I was funny, truthful, opinionated, and critical of all things I didn't understand in my narrow-minded thinking. Taking time to sit quietly and dive inwardly, I sighed in disbelief; complete shock took over my inner being when I realized that I had not been a good friend. I have been quite mean, abusive, and unloving to myself and everyone. Come to think of it, as a youth, I was always told I needed to acquire some tact . Never listening and only wanting to do things my way led me to think honesty was the best policy. This was my excuse for not thinking much about how I delivered my deadly words. Maybe this tough exterior developed from being the only girl and the middle child that was sometimes teased by my older brother. In my twenties, I heard the word *negative* used to describe my attitude toward life; by my forties, I was called obnoxious; during my marriage, I was frequently accused of being passive aggressive.

Becoming a good friend to myself would require me to give up all the comfortable habits that left me in a pity party and to let go of all the pretentious lies that led me further into a downward spiral. Wishing that my life would come to an end was not being a good friend to myself, but I found support in the social group of the Inner Fitness Project.

* * *

I woke up to the revelation that God did love me and knew that I was created for a purpose. You may be wondering how I arrived at this place of joy. The morning I woke up, words of negative intention did not resonate; I knew just how powerful my spoken words were in everything I was learning in the 14 Practices. They were all valuable to me, especially Practice 1—*I practice turning my life over to a power greater than me that loves me and responds to my heart. Greater* is the key expression of importance. This was hard to do. I was used to thinking I was in control of everything. Now, I look forward to waking up and try not to take my time on this planet for granted. As according to Practice 4—*I look for and work to transform the beliefs, patterns, and judgments I practice that limit my life*—I believe the universe is always communicating with me and shifting me to a greater awareness.

* * *

Every day is a journey to a better Self. The difference now is that I thirst for the connection of working the practices and being around the inspirational, like-minded individuals that are found in Practice 10. I cultivate social connections where I feel safe, seen, *and heard*. I believe there is a silver lining: My husband is truly alive through me. I stand in my truth and purpose not in the shadow of others. I have stopped comparing and worrying about what everyone else is doing. I am keeping my eyes on the prize of Self.

I can profoundly say working with Tina Lifford truly pushed me to believe in my dreams and more importantly the possibilities of my life. Thank you! It is my time to show God how much I truly love his universal presence.

Tianna: Getting Unstuck

STUCK. CHRONIC PROCRASTINATION. UNHEALTHY EATING. Self-hate. Isolation. Overweight. Anxiety. Depression. Loss of self. Loss of hope. Grieving being a parent to a special needs child. Unaware of goals/aspirations. Fear. Self-doubt. Always wishing things were better, but unsure of where to start.

That's where I was. My life had become a complete circle. Round and round, always ending back at the same point, and then repeating things over and over. If I tell myself the truth, I convinced myself that life would always be this way. I accepted this for myself, but deep down I wanted more, so although I was "used to it," it always felt like a fresh cut. I think the hardest thing for me to sit with was knowing that I needed to change, including knowing things I could do, but never following through with or committing to anything. It was tough because it just continued to feed my self-fulfilling prophesy that I was not good enough and didn't deserve a purposeful, divine, and fulfilled life.

Looking back over my life, I now realize that my childhood trauma was alive and well on my cyclical life journey. Abandonment by both my parents never allowed me to feel like I belonged to anything or anyone. It caused me to struggle with friendships and other relationships. In any relationship, I was never sure whether we were okay, and when there was ever a disagreement, I was sure and terrified that person would walk away. The wound that hurt the most, however, was the physical, emotional, and psychological abuse inflicted by my birth mother. This has caused me grave pain and crippled my growth. I could sit and rehash everything as if it had just happened, and that's what I hated the most. It lived in my memory like a present event. It was the foundation of my self-hate, self-judgment, and the big lies that felt like constant devastation. I recall thinking about my mother, *If she just dies, my life would be better*, and I saw nothing wrong with that. Not that I wanted to kill her, but if it happened at the hands of something or someone else, life would be so much better. It now makes me very sad to say this out loud, but my mind couldn't fathom any ounce of joy with her alive. I convinced myself that my joy, my purpose, and most important, my self-worth were wrapped up in my mother. That is the lie that pierced my heart like no other.

What ultimately led me to take the journey back to myself was that I began to become very angry and fed up with myself. I had had enough of my nonsense. At one point, it was like watching one of "those shows" where people need to get it together, but they keep doing the SAME thing and expecting different results. Imagine screaming "WHAT IS WRONG WITH YOU, GIRL?!?! STOP DOING THAT!"—but that girl is you. I became downright SICK of my unhealthy patterns. For so long I knew I needed to do better, but self-pity and victimization felt good and comfortable. Life was starting to become unhealthy, and all of a sudden, accountability, not harsh judgment, was creeping in! By this time, I was reading and had read so much that a little had crept in. The journey back to Self, as Tina always said, is constant work. I'm grateful that though I kept starting and stopping, the messages finally started to sink in. The knowledge that the universe is truly FOR and not against me has transformed my thinking. Knowing that something greater than me wants more for me, and most important, wants what I want for me, has been comforting and healing.

I discovered how powerful the mind truly is. I decided to try an experiment for one week. I told myself that no matter how hard things got, it was just life happening, and nothing personal against me. I told myself that if anything unpleasant came my way, I would just be grateful and ask the universe for help coping with it and for help not personalizing it. And you know what? That experiment had the AUDACITY to work. It worked! That's when I felt a shift. My mindset combined with understanding that the universe is *for* me, rather than against me, was the magic combo!

Well, I began testing it even more. I am most proud that my awareness was becoming sharper. I know it may seem small, but even waiting to be serviced in stores became a test. In the past, my patience had been paper thin, but now I began to wait with gratitude, and this shifted my mindset and also my energy. I told myself that sometimes you must wait. In the past I would say to myself, *I always get the line with the slow people*, and even just that thought allowed me to become the victim, once again. I am so aware now of how that mindset trickles into every minute of my day and every fiber of my being. The way people responded to me has been rewarding. Kind words. Smiles and gift cards for my patience. I mean, who doesn't love a Target gift card!

There has been a domino effect in so many areas of my life. Understanding that the universe loves me and is *for* me has changed the way I even parent. It has changed my language. I would always say, "I'm the mom of an autistic child." I would put that at the forefront of EVERYTHING. Again, self-victimization. Now I'm learning that this didn't happen *to* me. Some people have autism, and some don't. This is not to simplify or suggest that people with disabilities don't have challenges, but I realize now that operating from a place of grief and pity is different from advocating for and empowering my son. I'm no longer using his disability as my tragedy but realizing that he learns differently and I have to do things that may not be typical to raise him. That's really it. I did grieve the childhood I wanted for him, but the key word is *I*. I never took the time to sit and really pay attention to what *he* wanted. I am so aligned with my son now, and I am seeing how happy he has become without my silly limitations and mindset regarding who he is. I've realized that overachieving-despite is *my thing*. It has nothing to do with him. He is happy and delights in the things he loves. Being able to facilitate his happiness these past few weeks has been a joy I never knew I could have—a joy I never knew *we* could have. And I am so grateful.

I am finding myself living in the present. I am not beating myself up over old patterns that haven't served me. In the past I have struggled with weight and emotional eating, but I realize now that it was tied to the lie of me being unworthy. I was just keeping the lie alive in various ways. Now when I'm upset or happy, I reach for my journal instead of for food. I have started an Inner Fitness Workout regimen, and I am living in a space where I am grateful just to work out, instead of working out to get to a certain destination. I am living in the moment, daily, and leaving everything else where it belongs, in the past or in the future. Being this way decreases my chances of harmful self-judgment, all-or-nothing thinking, focusing on the past, and worrying about the future. I'm even providing space and grace for slipups. It has taken me decades to create and live with healthy habits and this mindset. Change will not happen overnight, but that doesn't mean change will not happen! I am ten pounds lighter, and every pound lost is a celebration! In the past I would downplay what seems little, but moving forward I work with the universe to celebrate everything. There are no big wins or little wins. There are wins, and lessons!

Where I am right now is intentionally setting my day. I no longer wake up with an attitude of "I hope this day will be okay." I wake up and claim my day, and I ask for understanding and help when things come that are out of my control. I have surrendered control of every aspect of my day. I do all things with gratitude so when things are unfavorable, I don't feel this all-or-nothing loss. I'm grateful for life and for the ability to experience good and bad.

Lately, feelings I thought were buried are resurfacing, and things are starting to hurt again. This is evidence that the walls around my heart are coming down and I am feeling once again. How good it is to *feel*! It's a part of the human experience I have missed. I know the hurt exists to inform me of those unhealed places. The universe is guiding me on what needs to heal, and for once, I am beyond appreciative and grateful for it. I am eating better, working out consistently, and finding new and creative ways to love on myself. My parenting is more patient, kind, and open-minded. I am daily letting go of expectations and allowing my son to be who he is, which is his birthright. I'm more consistent with my journey, and even when I don't do the things I know I should do, I don't judge myself harshly. I now hold myself accountable, lovingly.

Though it has taken me some time, I do not regret a thing. I genuinely believe I was meant to develop this greater sense of Self at this appointed time. My inner fitness journey has been authentic, genuine, and honest. Having an open mind to doing things differently was all the gas I needed to take off. What I love most about this journey, including the lovely soul I have become along the way, is that I feel no pressure to complete my healing by a certain time, nor do I feel the need to compete. This is a divine time in my life, and I have a solid understanding that this inner fitness journey is lifelong. I look forward to the ride!

In the future, I see me discovering things that I love! I can't WAIT to get to that part. My healing has thus far consisted of acknowledging old wounds and old lies and working to quiet my surviving self. Oh, to discover those little things that make my heart smile! I know they live inside me, but I look forward to discovering them so I can live them out loud! I realize now that locking down my heart locked me out of knowing who I truly am and what I enjoy in life. These things will allow me not only to cope, but to live life abundantly. In a nutshell, that's all I really want. I believe that by living abundantly I will discover and operate in my purpose. I know that I am a healer; I am here to help facilitate healing for others. I am eager to operate in my purpose because here I am healing myself, all because Tina said "yes" to her calling and is operating in her purpose!

I look forward to living a life that is in alignment with my higher Self. A life where the universe and I work together for the greater good. A life where I understand who I am and what I bring to the world. A life where I am not ignorant about hard times, but I won't allow them to make me forget how good life has been. A life where even if I stumble, I can always move forward. A life where I will be as kind to myself as I intentionally am with others. A life where I accept life in all its complexities and give myself much grace as I continue to navigate it.

Acknowledgments

We did it!

My deepest gratitude goes to Maura Mandell and Portia Flagg—for being so damn smart and true champions of the Inner Fitness Project mission; your care has made all the difference. Special thanks go to Frieda Lynn Morris, Deborah Stewart, and Darlene Hayes, for caring about this work and me. A heartfelt thank-you to family members Pam Lifford, Terra Lifford, and Chelsye Bernardez, who listened to me even when they were tired; I am blessed to have family that always shows up for one another. I am also blessed to have the heart and laser focus of the Inner Fitness Project COO and my friend, Morgan Stiff, who has the invaluable talent of seeing what's missing, and copywriter Krista Jones, who loves listening to and reading words. Dante Micheaux's love of language gave me the confidence to trust that my words matter. Friends Darlene Hayes and Deborah Stewart sharpened my focus.

Last but not least, I thank my editor, Patrik Bass, who has championed me from the moment we met, whose eye I can trust, and whose patience I appreciate. This is equally true of my agent, Johanna Castillo, who gets me and knows how to push when needed. And an excited thank-you goes to my publishing partners Judith Curr at HarperCollins and Viola Davis, Julius Tennon, and Lavaille Lavette at JVL.

About the Author

Tina Lifford's wisdom is her superpower. Often regarded as a modern-day mystic, Tina has spent over forty years mastering the art of spiritual and personal development. Her transformative Three Selves framework bridges the gap between a spiritual mindset and practical everyday application, making the path to inner freedom both accessible and empowering.

A passionate advocate for uplifting others, Tina is a licensed spiritual practitioner at Agape International Spiritual Center and an alumna of the University of Santa Monica Program in Spiritual Psychology. In addition to her online community and programs, she has served as an Inner Fitness educator at Georgia State University for the past four years and is actively involved in several women's organizations. Her previous book, *The Little Book of Big Lies*, was recognized as a *Forbes* must read in 2021.

In addition to her personal growth work, Tina is an award-winning actress. She has starred alongside legends such as Sidney Poitier, Clint Eastwood, and Bruce Willis, and has brought over one hundred characters to life on-screen.

Tina lives in Studio City, California, with her beloved dogs, Storm and Blu, and shares the role of family matriarch with her sister and best friend, Pam.

About Inner Fitness

The Inner Fitness Project and its community are a wellbeing movement. We are dedicated to making inner health and wellbeing (inner fitness) a lifestyle choice that is as well-understood, proactive, and actionable as physical fitness:

The Inner Fitness **Project** holds our mission.
The Inner Fitness **Studio** is our playground.
The Inner Fitness **Revolution** invites you to claim your right to thrive!

Our online community is committed to thriving through Self-awareness, effective tools, and the power of community. Discovering your whole Self is our #1 priority and passion. And we're damn good at it. Each offering meets you where you are and helps you grow into who you want to be. So you can invite your whole Self into every area of your life. Joyously. Authentically. Feeling full of possibilities.

Visit TheInnerFitnessProject.com for more information and to enroll in the revolutionary act of thriving unapologetically.